LISTENING CLOSELY

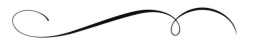

LISTENING CLOSELY
A Journey to Bilateral Hearing

ARLENE ROMOFF

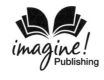

imagine!
Publishing

An Imagine Book
Published by Charlesbridge
85 Main Street
Watertown, MA 02472
617-926-0329
www.charlesbridge.com

Diagram on page 169 used by permission of Advanced Bionics LLC.
Book design by Cindy LaBreacht.

Library of Congress Cataloging-in-Publication Data

Romoff, Arlene.
    Listening closely : a journey to bilateral hearing / by Arlene Romoff.
        p. cm.
    Includes index.
    ISBN 978-1-936140-21-3 (reinforced for library use)
    ISBN 978-1-936140-22-0 (pbk.)
    1. Romoff, Arlene—Health. 2. Cochlear implants—Patients—United
States—Biography. 3. Directional hearing. I. Title.
RF305.R66 2010
617.8'820092—dc22
[B]
                                                        2010039255

Manufactured in China, November, 2010.

10 9 8 7 6 5 4 3 2 1

For information about custom editions, special sales,
premium and corporate purchases, please contact
Charlesbridge Publishing at specialsales@charlesbridge.com

TABLE OF CONTENTS

PREFACE

Opportunities to witness miracles in the making during one's career don't come along often, if at all. The cochlear implant, now widely used to treat severe to profound deafness in both adults and children, is just such a miracle. Reading this book, so aptly named, has convinced me how fortunate I've been to see this miracle unfold during my tenure.

I began practicing as an audiologist in 1979, before the first generation of multichannel cochlear implants existed for use in either children or adults. When a child was diagnosed with a profound sensorineural loss, or when an adult's progressive hearing loss reached the profound level, the one question asked by both parents and the deafened adult was, "Is there an operation that can help this type of hearing loss?" The answer was always no. As an audiologist I could offer powerful hearing aids, or refer my patients to the extensive resources of the League for the Hard of Hearing (now called the Center for Hearing and Communication) in New York City for speech and language therapy, to learn lipreading, to learn about assistive devices, and, very broadly, to learn how to live in the mainstream world as a deaf individual. I hoped that my advice and treatment recommendations were helpful, but I recognized only too well how imperfect they were, and the struggles that still remained for deaf children and adults alike. In fact, Arlene Romoff availed herself of these services—and her experiences, as detailed in this book, reflect this harsh reality.

The advent of the cochlear implant enabled audiologists and other hearing health care professionals to finally help minimize, in a most potent way, the struggles that our deaf clients face. Implants are not perfect; they do not restore hearing to normal, and each person's hearing history will impact how well they do. Yet, combined with an intensive, formal period of post-implant rehabilitation by qualified professionals, implants come closer to "perfecting" communication for our clients than we ever could have imagined.

I strongly believe that audiologists, speech-language pathologists, and otolaryngologists should read this book to get the insight they need to make them better able to serve their patients with severe to profound hearing loss who are facing the challenges Arlene describes. And, as did her first book, this volume will serve to help many people struggling with the decision of whether to get an implant, or a second implant. I think that after reading this book, the answer will be obvious.

But perhaps most significantly, even the casual reader will appreciate the experience of witnessing a true miracle in our lifetime— allowing people who are deaf to hear.

Laurie Hanin, PhD, CCC-A
Executive Director, Center for Hearing and Communication

PROLOGUE

Is life a series of random events that we react to? Or is there a grand design—a unifying thread that links moments to days to decades—with an intended purpose, a reason for us to be here? I've usually found myself too occupied going from event to event to even think about it. I've always tried to have some good come of life's trials and tribulations—not just picking myself up and coping, but helping others along the way: basically, "making lemons into lemonade." I thought I had perfected this to a fine art, even attaining some "wisdom of age." It seemed to be a fulfilling philosophy, giving shape and reason to all I had encountered in my many years on earth. That is, until March 3, 2008. But I had better start from the beginning, since any talk about a grand design is all in the details, anyway.

I was born with normal hearing, which enabled me to develop normal speech and socialization skills. It wasn't until my late teens that my hearing began to slip. I got through college and started my job as a computer programmer without much problem. But by age twenty-three, I had to get my first hearing aid. My hearing continued to decline slowly, going through mild, moderate, severe, and profound levels of loss over the next twenty-five years. There was never any reason given for this degenerative loss, but it was a devastating experience. I had to continually keep up with new hearing aids, assistive listening equipment, and lipreading skills just to function during this depressing and chaotic downward spiral.

My personal philosophy to make the most of whatever situation I found myself in resulted in my becoming an ardent advocate for people with hearing loss. Because of my long, slow descent into deafness, I developed into quite an expert on coping strategies at every level. My advocacy work also encompassed getting assistive listening systems and captioning provided in public places—essential accommodations for people with hearing loss, myself included.

I eventually lost virtually all of my hearing, finally confronting that word: *deaf*. Hearing aids were of no use to me any longer. It was then that I opted to get a cochlear implant (CI). Cochlear implants use electrodes threaded into the cochlea, an internal computer chip, and an external computer processor to bypass the damaged portion of the cochlea and stimulate the auditory nerve directly, allowing sound to reach the brain. There should be no doubt in anyone's mind that cochlear implants are a modern miracle, enabling the deaf to hear.

I was no pioneer when I got my CI in 1997, but so few people knew about what CIs could do that I set about educating others— professionals and people with hearing loss—about the miracle of this technology. I chronicled the first year with my CI, which became the basis for my book, *Hear Again: Back to Life with a Cochlear Implant*. With that book, I achieved my goal of helping others by relating my own experiences and advice. I was particularly touched by the heartfelt expressions of thanks I received from people who benefitted from this information. I thought that as more people got CIs, the world would embrace this technology and realize that true miracles are still possible here on earth. I was wrong.

I had my CI for over ten years, upgrading the external hardware and software as much as possible as the technology improved. Even though many more children and adults were getting them, the mainstream population, including doctors who were not ear specialists, still had no idea what CIs were all about. I would invariably hold a normal conversation with a hearing person, telling them that I was totally deaf and hearing them with my CI, and they would ask me, "And does that device help you?" How could they not be aware of what it means to be deaf and the enormity of this miracle? It just didn't make any sense!

I continued to help people through my advocacy and outreach efforts, and I came to believe that was my mission in life—just as others have career goals. I was certainly comfortable with the idea. When I would plaintively ask, "Why me?" the answer was always, "Why not?" I could even grasp the bigger picture of having to endure twenty-five years of degenerative hearing loss before being "rescued" by my CI. I accepted that as the necessary on-the-job training for my life's work.

I was in no rush to "go bilateral," though, getting another CI in my other ear. I was functioning rather well, I thought, and I had reacted so poorly to the anesthesia of my CI surgery that I didn't want to endure that again. I was content to be a one-sided user of ten-year-old CI technology, no matter what the shortcomings.

Everything about my life that I've described so far seemed to be driven by my responses to everyday events. Some things were fortuitous, some not, but the direction was always clear—make the most of what life dished out. But now I'm in a quandary about how to describe the events that transformed my life. In one year, I went from being a user of ten-year-old CI technology in one ear to a person with state-of-the art CI technology in both ears. In the process, I also produced a chronicle documenting this metamorphosis, which is contained in these pages. For all this to happen, however, my first implant had to stop working, I had to have it surgically replaced, and then have yet another surgery to implant the other ear. I also needed a support network to help carry me through this unexpected odyssey. How these events unfolded, and the circumstances surrounding them, were often ironic, too perfect, coincidental, or impeccably timed. Incredibly, often "things happened" that served to soften the stresses and rigors of this transition. How else to explain why my old CI stopped working at a CI support group meeting or how I learned the day before my surgery that I could have a trained hearing loss specialist actually hold my hand in the operating room? Chance?

For some people, the words *too perfect* or *coincidental* indicate some degree of religious faith or divine intervention. For others who don't have these beliefs, they would be construed just as described and nothing more. Personally, I do sense a grand design—something beyond individual events or occurrences.

I'm reminded of the note cards I won as a door prize at an event at my temple the very first year I had my CI. Pictured on the front was a nautilus shell, which is shaped like a cochlea, with the inscription LISTEN CLOSELY. I had always thought those cards were a little "too perfect," and I've pondered their significance ever since.

It does seem that these life-changing events are part of some elaborate plan. Taking a broad perspective, it seems that with a single ten-year-old CI in one ear, I had outlived my usefulness to counsel others on current CI technology and practices. This was remarkably similar to my situation in 1997, when my first CI came along just as my hearing reached a level that was so poor I could no longer function. In both cases, state-of-the-art technology enabled me to continue my advocacy work. The timing, once again, was exactly right, with a curious convergence of circumstances. My medical insurance company had just started covering bilateral CIs in the past year. The ten-year warranty on my CI had just expired, so even though most CIs last far longer than that, it wouldn't be considered a "premature failure." Most of the shortcomings of my first CI—noise, distance, music—are now addressed by the latest technology, and having CIs in both ears would mitigate the limitations of listening with one ear alone. And there's no ignoring the fact that my first book, while still useful in many respects, is lacking in current information.

But there's also that unfinished business of finally recognizing CIs as the miracle they are. A ten-year-old device in one ear that enables the deaf to hear is still a miracle, but it's the latest information about the benefits of bilateral CIs—and how their interaction with the brain brings hearing even closer to normal—that is the miracle that needs to be broadcast *now*. And what can deliver that message? It does seem that this book is destined for the task.

Whether everyone would agree that there is some grand design at play here is not really my concern. Reflecting on my forty-year odyssey with hearing loss, I realize now that there were events and responses that clearly shaped my future. In the span of a year, however, the circumstances have been unmistakable. The opportunities and problems presented to me practically dared me to make the most of them, along with enigmatic signposts that were ironic, too perfect, or coincidental. Whether this indicates some sort of divine intervention, or just chance, I will leave for you to decide.

Whatever your beliefs, you cannot truly appreciate the enormity of enabling the deaf to hear without fully understanding the impact of deafness on daily living. On the following pages, you will walk in my shoes. For those with hearing loss, and parents of children with hearing loss, I hope you will benefit from my adventures using new technology and hearing with two ears. For those with normal hearing, I hope you'll envision yourself in my world, so you can finally grasp—with appropriate awe—exactly why a device that enables the deaf to hear is truly a miracle of Biblical proportions.

Listen closely . . .

LAYING THE
FOUNDATION

From Normal to Deaf
in Twenty-five Years

M ost people don't give much thought to hearing. It is invisible and happens without any effort if it is working right. It is hard to imagine what it would be like *not* to hear. You can close your eyes or try out a wheelchair to simulate other disabilities, but trying to replicate a hearing loss is far more elusive. Most people don't realize how much a loss of hearing can impact daily living until they experience it themselves. Then it is an eye-opener.

I was like that. I was born with normal hearing, just like everyone else in my family. My parents were high school instrumental music teachers, so my world was filled with music—classical music. My father always listened to WQXR broadcasts on his hi-fi radio, and I'm sure I absorbed symphonies and sonatas without even realizing it. My vocabulary was sprinkled with words like *pizzicato*, *vibrato*, and *Scheherazade*.

I didn't have any problems with my hearing growing up, although I do recall thinking that I could "hear silence." That must have been tinnitus, an early indication that something was wrong. I began piano lessons at age eight, and played in many recitals. The European piano teachers at the Third Street Music School in New York City would tell me I looked just like a French painting—and years later, I discovered that I did resemble some of Renoir's portrait children, with my auburn hair. I continued my piano studies, taking up the oboe as well, and got through high school without a problem. Ironically, my first realization that something wasn't right with my hearing was when my piano no longer sounded in tune. I was losing my sense of pitch.

I got through four years of college and was married a year later. I heard my wedding vows perfectly—"in sickness and in health." Little did I suspect the years of declining hearing that lay ahead, with my husband, Ira, now destined to be my companion on this journey. Our first dance was "Someone to Watch Over Me."

Just a year later, when I was on the job as a computer programmer, I knew I needed hearing aids. My inability to hear well impacted virtually every activity. My world was crashing in on me as a result of something that most people—hearing people—can never fully understand: the life-changing impact of even a moderate hearing loss.

It turned out that I had a fluctuating degenerative hearing loss, which was frustratingly difficult to fit with a hearing aid. My first audiologist gave up on me and referred me to the League for the Hard of Hearing (now called the Center for Hearing and Communication). Ironically, what I initially thought was a hopeless situation turned out to be the best thing that ever happened to me. The League was exactly the right place to be because they focused on functioning. It took two full years for them to fit me with a hearing aid. But I also took lipreading classes and learned all about the assistive listening devices available to help me function better, making up for the limitations of my hearing aid. I needed all the help I could get, too. By then, I had two children who were depending on me! I needed to be proactive about my own communication needs, not only for myself, but because I was fending for my children, too. "Shy little Arlie" turned into tenacious but polite "Don't-Mess-with-Me Arlene." I couldn't be shy with a hearing loss. I learned that if I was upfront and honest, people would usually respond with understanding and consideration.

The operative word for a degenerative hearing loss is always *less*, and the sounds of my world grew silent one by one. Keys stopped jingling, acorns no longer crunched underfoot, and even the footsteps themselves were finally hushed. Holidays and annual events became benchmarks of this incessant decline. Instead of happy occasions, they were depressing reminders that I heard less than the year before.

Hearing tests were equally traumatic, with the added insult of having numbers attached to those assessments, and tissues were de rigueur to catch the tears of despair. The quest for stronger hearing aids, assistive listening equipment, and better lipreading skills was constant, with the hearing loss always one step ahead of functioning. One little gadget that helped me stay connected far longer than I might have was a small auxiliary microphone that plugged directly into my hearing aid. I held it up to people's mouths interview style, getting as much usable sound as possible while lipreading the rest.

The daily impact of a degenerative hearing loss could be described as psychological torture. An ever-growing wall of isolation kept me from communicating freely with those around me. I was cut off from the mainstays of our culture—music, movies, and socialization. Conversation, even when I was included, focused on important information—never anything incidental, which wasn't worth the energy needed to comprehend it. If I missed understanding something, I was told all too often that it was "not important." Without audible cues, I was always on high alert, using my eyes to make up for my ears. Even trying my hardest to stay in communication, it was inevitably not enough, and in the end I always felt "beaten up."

I developed carefully honed coping skills—not necessarily to improve communication, but just to survive without humiliation in social settings. I perfected the art of the "manipulated conversation" —a calculated strategy in which I would set the topic of conversation, ask questions that I didn't need to know the answers to, and appear to be charming and intelligent without ever having to understand a word the other person was saying. Needless to say, this was an exhausting exercise during which I learned absolutely nothing about the person I was talking to, but it got me through social situations with my dignity intact. I also learned the art of the "joyless smile," the one I trotted out when I had no idea what was going on.

I considered most social events cruel and unusual punishment—not surprising when considering the effort required just to appear "normal." Even mundane occurrences such as an elevator's *ding*, bakery numbers being called, and casual comments by store clerks, flight attendants, or even toll collectors, were fraught with anxiety and dread when they couldn't be heard.

I was raised Jewish, and although I wasn't strictly observant, I did have my own perspectives on God and faith. Praying for my hearing to return, however, was not even a realistic possibility then. All I humbly wanted was the strength to deal with this challenge. From the first days, that is what I prayed for, knowing full well that the act of prayer itself tapped an inner strength.

I also took very seriously the commandment to "do mitzvot," generally translated as doing good deeds. At that point in my life, when I was seeking solutions, I felt that whatever I learned could also be helpful to others. The impact of hearing loss on my life was so bewildering, with so few good answers, I knew that others must be floundering in this netherworld as well.

When the Americans with Disabilities Act (ADA) was signed into law in 1991, I became a founding member of the League's volunteer advocacy committee, Advocates for Better Communication. That plunged me into advocacy for real! 1991 was also the year my hearing became too poor to use a regular voice telephone. Coincidentally, that was the same year that the Federal Communications Commission (FCC) mandated that every state must have its own Telecommunications Relay Service. Relay allowed Teletype (TTY) phone users to make calls to regular phone users, with the text of their speech transcribed by an operator. My friend, who had never been able to use a regular phone, told me how lucky I was to have lost my hearing at that time, and to have Relay available to me. Somehow I didn't feel lucky, but in retrospect, I guess I was, because it allowed me to communicate by phone and pursue my advocacy work. The Internet and e-mail would come later.

My advocacy efforts focused on my needs, which may sound selfish, but I knew that if I needed something, so would many other people with hearing loss. I enjoyed going to the theater, but that, too, was becoming a frustrating experience because I could no longer hear most of the dialogue, even with the assistive listening devices theaters provided. I was desperate not to lose yet another of life's pleasures, and the captioning of live theater performances became my passion. It made sense to me that if a theater could provide sign language interpreters in front of a section of the audience, they could easily put the text up there as well. Working with a court reporter and other "hearing angels," the equipment and logistics were ultimately worked out. The first open captioned performances debuted at the Paper Mill Playhouse in New Jersey in 1996 with *Gigi*, and on Broadway in 1997 with *Barrymore*, a one-man show starring Christopher Plummer. I had virtually no hearing left on that historic evening and couldn't even converse using my little auxiliary microphone. In spite of that, it was a wonderful theater experience. Although I heard very little, I didn't miss a word of the dialogue. It was an incredible feeling knowing that, because of *my* efforts, so many people were able to enjoy a show they wouldn't have attended otherwise.

The timing of this artistic triumph was ironic as well. My advocacy efforts, which were fueled by my declining hearing and my mission to help others, had delivered open captioned live theater to the masses just as I was poised to get my first cochlear implant. My surgery was scheduled for the following month and marked the end of my twenty-five-year descent from normal hearing to profound deafness.

Cochlear Implants— Surgery and Activation

A cochlear implant is composed of two parts—an internal component, which must be surgically inserted, and an external processor, which is a dedicated microcomputer. Many people think that cochlear implant surgery actually fixes something in the ear, but its sole objective is to place a computer chip and magnet under the scalp and thread an electrode array into the cochlea. The external processor interfaces with the internal component at the magnet site, picking up sounds with its external microphone and sending signals via radio waves through the scalp to the computer chip, which controls the firing of the electrodes in the cochlea, stimulating the auditory nerve directly, which is then perceived by the brain as sound. The external processor fits either behind the ear like a hearing aid, or is worn on the body like a beeper. (See diagram on page 169.)

My first cochlear implant surgery was in October 1997 and was done under general anesthesia, taking about two and a half hours. It encompassed some drilling of bone to insert the electrode array into the cochlea and position the computer chip and magnet under the scalp. I didn't have much pain after the procedure, and found that Tylenol was sufficient. I did, however have a poor reaction to the anesthesia, which made me hyperactive for three weeks after the surgery. Thankfully, that didn't interfere with my activation date, which was scheduled for the following week.

The activation of the processor—hearing my first sounds—was an incredible event! The external device had to be programmed by my audiologist, a process called *mapping*. She hooked my processor up to a computer and I had to determine comfortable volume levels of several pitches, which she then used to create a program. The device was then turned on, and I listened to her speak, using that program. At my very first mapping session, I had been warned that those first sounds would be weird and electronic, that it would take the brain a while to adapt—and this turned out to be true. Even so, I was still able to discern speech right away. How one adapts to a cochlear implant, however, is very individual. One's hearing history, length of deafness, and age at onset of deafness have a major impact on the entire adaptation process. As a late-deafened adult who once had normal hearing, I was expected to do well right away—and I did.

It's important to realize that using a cochlear implant is not like putting on glasses. It takes time for the brain to adapt to perceiving sounds with the device, and every cochlear implant user quickly becomes aware that it is a "brain thing." While it would seem that each mapping session should lead to big improvements in hearing, the reality is that the brain adapts slowly and change happens gradually. Mappings are scheduled every few weeks, as the brain's perception of sound changes and matures. What can start out as very robotic-sounding speech gradually becomes more natural with time.

It's quite an odyssey to experience the brain in action, and many cochlear implant users start referring to their brains as if they were separate entities—and in a way they are. The first main challenge for the brain is to process the sounds it is hearing and interpret them as words—speech. To speed this process along, auditory rehabilitation is usually recommended. For me, that meant listening to books on tape (back in 1997, there were no CD or MP3 players). I was able to understand the words without following along with the text, something not all CI users can do right away. This method also trained my brain to rely on listening, and not on visual cues—a hard habit to break!

I am probably making the cochlear implant process sound a little too simple. The reality is that the computer technology driving this system is enormously complex and sophisticated. How the software can interface with the microcomputer to allow the brain to perceive speech, and even music, by stimulating parts of the auditory nerve thousands of times per second, is mind-boggling. And the other equally important half of this equation—how the brain adapts—is almost incomprehensible. The brain gets better at hearing with time, practice, and patience, and its perception of sound can actually evolve, even if no programming changes are made. It is no wonder I continue to believe that the most appropriate description of this process is *miracle*.

Capabilities and Limitations

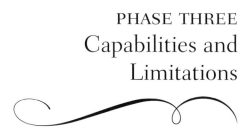

My first days, weeks, and even months after that initial activation were filled with awe and wonder. Yet right before my CI was activated, I doubted whether I really would be able to hear again—it was too incredible to imagine. When my world actually did come alive again, it was as though the sound track had been added to my silent movie! I could even use a regular phone again. The revelation of hearing sounds was just the beginning, though.

Hearing loss is a communications disability, and I had been cut off from people. A hearing person can't possibly imagine what this is like, other than to realize that the worst punishment given to prisoners is usually solitary confinement. Being put back into the world of social interactions wasn't just a matter of turning the sound back on. Having the confidence to interact with others had to be relearned.

That first year with my CI was one of rediscovery. Human beings were designed to talk to one another. I was intrigued by the little pleasantries I heard daily from people in shops, the bank, or the post office: "Have a nice day," or, "Enjoy it." Most hearing people think this idle chatter is unimportant, but those words connect people to one another. Imagine not being able to hear those verbal smiles—or worse, wondering what those people were saying.

And my name! Imagine hearing your name for the first time in decades—and finally having a reason to use it! I no longer had to be touched or jabbed to get my attention. "Arlene." I hear you!

After only a few weeks, I came to realize that my friends and my family were as eager to talk to me as I was to hear them. I had always been so focused on trying to lipread and communicate that it never occurred to me that the isolation my deafness imposed actually went both ways. It prevented people from talking to me—and I learned that they wanted to!

I found myself not only welcoming human contact, but seeking it out. I started initiating conversations, something I never would have done—and never *could* have done—with a profound hearing loss. This didn't happen automatically just because I could hear again. It took time to adapt, not only to hearing speech again, but also to the subtle social behaviors that go along with oral communication. I was gradually coming out of my shell.

The impact of deafness is often insidious, taking its toll on self-confidence and self-esteem. After almost a year with my CI, I felt that I was finally behaving like a "real person." Imagine the social deprivation that would result in that kind of assessment! The adaptation was ongoing, well beyond that first year, with not only my hearing improving, but also my self-confidence. It had, after all, taken twenty-five years to sink from normal hearing into deafness, so it would take some time to realize that this sudden reversal wasn't a dream. I became more gregarious as my self-confidence grew, and I realized that, for the first time in decades, my hearing was actually improving!

I wasn't naive, though. I understood that my hearing was still not normal, but how could I possibly complain about that? I had just been rescued from solitary confinement! It was still a miracle, even if it wasn't perfect! I figured out that there were environments I did better in, and some where I did worse. It all boiled down to the noise level and the distance from the speech source. I functioned best speaking to someone who was close to me in a quiet environment. As either the distance or the noise level increased, I found it increasingly difficult to hear.

As I continued to use my CI, my ability to hear *did* improve, and that included music. I enjoyed listening to most kinds of music, both vocal and instrumental. The one instrument that remained most elusive was the organ. It actually took two years before I could hear that accurately—it had sounded like electronic mush up until then.

I upgraded to a behind-the-ear processor in 2001, replacing my beeper-sized model, and that brought some improved functioning, particularly in noise. That processor also had limitations, but there was no way for me to predict how well I would ultimately hear with it. With hearing in only one ear, I was very "one-sided" and it was hard to converse with people who weren't on my "good side." That also made it difficult to know where sounds were coming from—directionality. I wasn't upset or ungrateful. I hoped that I would continue to do better as time went on. I always likened this process to painting a masterpiece, and one doesn't rush a masterpiece.

Noisy restaurants remained my most difficult environment, and ironically, I wrote what turned out to be a most prescient statement in my book, *Hear Again*:

"I really want to be able to converse with people on both sides of me, and also across the table. Boy, do I set tough standards! Well, if we are going for miracles, then let's go for them!"

That was an interesting wish, because I never was able to function with ease in a noisy restaurant with my first CI processor, not in the ten years that I used it. It would ultimately take improved technology and two ears to accomplish that. There wasn't a day, however, that I didn't consider my hearing a miracle. When the *New York Times* printed an article about cochlear implants in its *Science* section on Tuesday, February 26, 2008, I jumped at the opportunity to shout to the world my continued awe at being able to hear again. I wrote:

"As a cochlear implant user for the past ten years, I am still in awe of being able to hear again, and reminded daily of its enormous impact on my quality of life. I doubt that hearing people will ever truly grasp the magnitude of this miracle."

I e-mailed that letter to the *Times* on Thursday, February 28 and heard back from them two days later, informing me that it was likely to be printed in the next *Science* section. Inexplicably, my cochlear implant stopped working the next day.

My metamorphosis had begun . . .

TRANSFORMATION

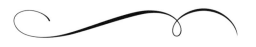

Twenty-four Days of Silence

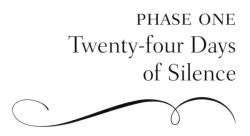

Sunday, March 3 began routinely. I was on the computer, then on the phone, talking for a half hour with my friend. Everything was fine, no inkling of anything wrong. I went to do my hair, taking off my CI processor, and when I put it back on, there was no sound. I didn't panic because the problem could be the battery, the connecting cable, the microphone, or even the external processor. I had replacement parts for these components and tried them all. There was still no sound. That meant the problem had to lie with the internal component, and there was no quick fix for that, only surgical replacement.

I panicked and burst into tears.

My husband Ira heard my shrieks and came running. We went through everything again. Still silence—deaf silence. At least I could lipread my husband with no sound, so we weren't cut off from communicating with each other. It was just so much more difficult than hearing. We weren't quite sure where to go, though. We were in Florida, not our home base in New Jersey. We called the CI company and they gave us the name of an audiology practice that could troubleshoot my processor problems.

We had an appointment the next day, and in those twenty-four hours, my disposition went from panic to bitter impatience. The audiologist was wonderful and understanding. She was in touch with the CI company's hotline audiologist and we tried various combinations of new processors and cords, all to no avail. She was determined not to give up and gave it one last try—a different body-worn processor model and headpiece. Incredibly, that made a connection, and as I turned up the volume, I was hearing again! But we all knew that I was hanging by a thread. The computer showed that I shouldn't be hearing, but I was. We made an appointment with the CI company's audiologist to do an official assessment one week later. I came home in a quasi-trance, happy to be connected again, but not knowing how long it would last.

With all the hubbub, I had almost forgotten about my letter to the *New York Times.* I checked their website before going to bed and, sure enough, there it was. My letter exclaiming the enormous impact my cochlear implant had on my quality of life was now staring back at me from my computer—and from Tuesday's *Science* section of the print version as well. Those words meant so much to me when I wrote them. They were practically shouting at me now!

Reality started to sink in. I didn't even have a CapTel phone here, the kind that provides the text of a phone conversation for people who can't hear well. I had left mine in New Jersey, never thinking that I'd need it. The next day, March 5, provided an interesting turn of events, though. After years of deliberating, the FCC finally approved a service called WebCapTel, which enables a person to use a regular telephone and a computer screen to function like a CapTel phone. I no longer needed an actual CapTel phone to have my phone calls captioned! I thought the impeccable timing of this announcement was a little bizarre, and it made me even more certain that my processor was destined to go silent again. I just didn't know when.

The conventional wisdom when confronting challenging situations is to take one day at a time, and the next day didn't disappoint. On March 6, the only known photo of Helen Keller holding a doll surfaced after being hidden in an album for the past 120 years. It had been taken in 1888, when Helen was eight years old, and was significant because *doll* was one of the first words she learned. But a picture of a girl holding a doll was significant to me as well. I collect dolls, and I also collect pictures of girls with their dolls—not just any pictures, but photos known as *cabinet cards*, which were popular in the 1880s. It had also become customary for my family to give me dolls instead of flowers when I was sick or in the hospital. To have this photo emerge after 120 years during the week that I was tottering on the brink of deafness—was this my get-well gift?

I showed Ira the photo and told him about its history, and even he gasped. He was always on the lookout for lovely girl-with-doll themed items for me, whether pictures or figurines. He had always been the one to tell others to "get Arlene dolls, not flowers" when I was recuperating from my various surgeries. For this photograph to emerge now, after 120 years—that was a bit much to comprehend. I had no choice but to keep going, though. One day at a time was becoming my mantra.

My processor was still working that Saturday night, March 8, so we kept our plans to see a George Gershwin revue at a local theater. Of course, one of the featured songs was "Someone to Watch Over Me," the music we first danced to at our wedding—all too appropriate now.

I had promised my friend Andrea that I would go with her to a local CI support group meeting the next day. I was having second thoughts about going, considering the precarious nature of my hearing, but I didn't want to disappoint her, so we kept our plans. We sat together at the meeting and waited our turns to introduce ourselves. At the precise moment that Andrea finished speaking and handed me the microphone, my processor stopped working—dead silence. The split-second timing was impeccable, perfectly choreographed. But if there were any place that could be considered a "soft landing," that was it. I was sitting in a room full of the most understanding people in the world—other cochlear implant users.

I should have been overcome with tears and emotion, but I wasn't. For some reason I was able to lipread Andrea, and she kept making me laugh. I guess they send angels to supervise these soft landings.

The next day was my appointment with the CI company's audiologist. Ira accompanied me. We knew what the verdict was going to be, so it wasn't a surprise when my internal component was officially pronounced dead. My reaction was almost blasé. I had already run the gamut of emotions and had nothing left.

What could we do now? We went to the movies—a captioned movie. My advocacy the previous month had ensured that a local theater would show captioned movies all the time, so we went, happy to think about something other than hearing. We had our work cut out for us, though, setting up the doctor and hospital appointments for the "revision" surgery.

There was one significant problem, however—a situation I had never resolved. The surgeon who had done my original surgery was no longer at the New York University Medical Center, but the audiologist who had programmed my CI all these years still was. I wasn't sure what to do since the surgeon and audiologist usually work in tandem. The decision about where to have the surgery was weighing on me. I didn't want to slight my original surgeon, who was wonderful, well-known, and respected. Ira called his office, but it was closed for two weeks. They were in the process of moving, so it was impossible to make any appointments with them. The timing, once again, was impeccable. I needed an appointment now. There was no decision to be made—it had been made for me. I would stay at NYU for my surgery and audiological follow-up. Ira made the pre-op doctor and hospital appointments and scheduled the surgery date: March 28. We were good to go—almost! We still hadn't heard back from Betsy Bromberg, my audiologist, about an activation date when I would be returned to sound. We knew she had to shuffle appointments to accommodate me, but we figured we would hear from her eventually.

Being plunged into silence was proving to be even more traumatic than I had expected. My body tensed up and would not calm down. We had to cancel all social engagements with friends. There was no point in seeing them if I couldn't hear. I could lipread Ira, but it was becoming too strenuous to converse freely. I was trying to keep a good attitude, but my mind started to lose focus. I was definitely feeling the effects of "solitary confinement."

After five days of silence, I was searching for some sense of order in the chaotic thoughts swirling through my mind. I was beginning to lose it. I began to write. I needed to write.

MARCH 14, 2008 What I've Learned So Far— Five Days without Sound

Being without sound after having a cochlear implant for ten years— the best description that comes to mind is purgatory. It's impossible to function like a human being, simply because human beings talk to one another, and without hearing, that's pretty much impossible.

Purgatory may be a harsh description, but it does imply that it's preparation for a better place. It's not hell, but it's not earth, either, because there's too much here on earth that can't be done without hearing. But that's not to say that one can't have a good attitude and still be in this situation. It just demands that the reality of what one can do and what one can't do be faced honestly and rationally.

The most problematic area is in-person communication because speech-to-speech requires lipreading on the part of the person without sound. This can be immensely exhausting if done at the same pace and duration as when there was sound. The irony is that the people closest to the person without sound bear the brunt of this situation. It's best to realize this early on, to avoid the exhaustion of trying to maintain "normalcy." Dealing with this in a rational manner should ideally take the emotion out of it so requests to curtail conversation aren't taken personally.

Figuring out what activities are not impacted by lack of hearing is the best way to go. If I were a golfer, heading out to the driving range would make a lot of sense. But I prefer a walk through nature—a garden, park, or beach.

Any activity that brings one close to other people is bound to result in someone trying to make conversation, which you won't understand unless your lipreading is superb, which mine is not. Being prepared in advance should remove the anxiety.

Smiling and saying that your hearing aids are being repaired is one way to gracefully exit such awkward moments. The sad part of this situation is that it is denying a very basic human trait—interacting with other humans. But the stress of trying to do this just isn't worth the struggle or effort. It's probably best to content oneself with exchanging smiles. At least that's a form of human communication—and smiling can be therapeutic in itself.

Given some thought, I'm sure there are other activities—usually done solo—that can be pleasant and that don't rely on hearing. Staying hopeful that this is a temporary situation should provide the strength to keep going. Fortunately, I don't have to worry about functioning on a job or taking care of young children—enormous challenges without hearing.

Anything visual is usually good. In the case of communication via language, that would mean text—books, e-mail, instant messages, text messaging, captioned television, captioned movies, captioned theater. All of these work as ways to keep connected to other human beings, and also as substitutes for the mental stimulation that is lacking because of the absence of sound.

One activity that can be done, hearing or not, is crying. And while that may be construed as giving in to pity or not having a good attitude, it's a human activity. And if it relieves stress, and it feels good to be able to do something that is "normal," then that's okay, too.

WRITING THIS DOWN felt good, a therapeutic exercise to preserve my sanity, but I realized it was an opportunity as well—to document, in real time, the experience of being plunged into silence. Writing about it in hindsight would not capture the raw emotions.

We still hadn't heard from Betsy with an activation date, though, and Ira thought we should call her. I was working on a crossword puzzle at the time—an activity I could do without hearing—and stopped cold after filling in the letters to 23-Across. "HEAVENS TO BETSY" was the answer. Somehow I didn't think we were going to have to call

Betsy. I checked my e-mail, and there was her message waiting for me, along with the activation appointment information—April 2 and 3.

I really didn't know what to think anymore, except that I knew I had to keep writing. I was no longer writing just to help myself get through this. It was now apparent to me that I would be writing to help others who might encounter sudden deafness and also to educate others about what it is like to live in silence like this. And so my "days without sound" continued . . .

MARCH 18, 2008 What I've Learned So Far— Nine Days without Sound

Nine days into this odyssey, and the initial shock to my system of not hearing is starting to let up. I no longer have intense physical feelings of agitation and tenseness, but the stress is still there. Nothing is normal; everything is on high alert, déjà vu of how things used to be prior to my implant. Vigilance must replace sound reception, and that produces a unique stress of its own. The result is that I have no buffer zone to cushion life's little nuisances. All my emotions and responses are close to the surface; there is no calm.

Unique is an apt description for this entire situation. How to explain ten years of functioning in a world full of sound and then being plunged into silence, accompanied only by relentless cacophonous tinnitus? (Today's selection is organ dissonance with an occasional helicopter landing.) This is not the same deafness I came from before. Then, I hadn't known sound for so long, I literally didn't realize what I was missing. But this—this is something entirely different, a challenge to overcome, a time warp to live through as best I can. The saving grace is that if all goes according to plan, there will be an end, and I will return to what has been "normal" for me for the past ten years.

Lipreading without sound continues to be the most difficult of challenges. All in-person communication is reliant on this, making communication with my husband most difficult. I had never really done lipreading without sound before, except for the few moments I'd have my CI off before going to sleep or in a beauty salon. It's exhausting work to lipread this way, and by the end of the day, it is simply too much. My brain shuts down and effectively says, "We're not doing this anymore!" I can't blame it—lipreading is an imprecise art because only 30 percent of speech sounds show up on the lips, making it a creative exercise to figure out the other 70 percent. Sounds such as *H*, *G*, and *K* don't show up at all, and it suddenly seems as if my husband's entire vocabulary is centered on words using those letters! Coupled with stress and a short temper, it's a volatile combination. It doesn't seem as though lipreading should be so exhausting, so mere explanations aren't convincing. It was only when I responded to Ira without voice—without him understanding a word—that he understood what I was dealing with. We've discovered that S-L-O-W-E-R is definitely better, trying not to distort the words, but giving the brain more time to process the input.

One plus—if we can call it that—is that people from all parts of my life have been offering words and gestures of love, caring, and support. Hearing from people via e-mail has been heartening, and so welcome, especially because in-person communication has become so impossibly difficult. Many of these people know me because of my first book, *Hear Again—Back to Life with a Cochlear Implant,* and it is so meaningful to know that what I wrote seems to have touched so many. One person, offering his best wishes on my upcoming surgery, pulled up the e-mail exchange we had seven years ago, when discussing my book. I would never have imagined that happening, which is why I'm having new thoughts and perspectives about this entire ordeal.

I also received a very touching and supportive e-mail from another CI user, expressing hope that my time without sound would go quickly. Oddly enough, I was very troubled by that sentiment. I really don't want to wish away a part of my life! I can understand the times in our lives when we are in such pain—either physically or emotionally—that we'd like to fast forward to be done with it. But as troubling as this entire situation is, it simply doesn't rise to that level of severity. But, take careful note—that's taking into consideration this huge leap of faith that, at the end, I will have my hearing back!

My feeling is that this is a challenge, and it's something that I'll learn from, hopefully cope with the best I can, and it too will be part of the tapestry of my life. If my brain can create symphonies from the input of sixteen electrodes, surely it can be coaxed into thinking that a month without sound is a great adventure! My brain is still not at all convinced, but as the days continue to pass, it is coming around a bit.

My children have made a concerted effort to e-mail and instant message me more frequently, to make up for the lack of phone and in-person human contact. Just the other day, my son IMed me, and since he and I share a sense of humor that I would characterize as "genetic," we had an incredible, hysterical, funny exchange that had me laughing so convulsively, I had to save it on my computer and print it out. It is *still* making me laugh just thinking about it!

Now, could this have happened if everything had been as before —no CI failure and communication as always? Maybe, but I doubt it. That made me think, and maybe my brain took note as well, that this could be an adventure—surely not one that I or anyone else would have chosen, but one that could possibly expose new insights, experiences, and perhaps even wisdom.

This immediately brought to mind my daughter Emily's shell-collecting habits along the beaches of the Gulf coast many years ago. She always picked up broken shells, and when I asked her why, she looked at me curiously because the answer was so obvious to her. They were beautiful. She saw the beauty even in broken shells and, by extension, others around her that weren't perfect. She showed me her favorite—a spiral, or cochlea-shaped, shell that was so broken you could see the inner helix. She pointed out that you'd never be able to see that wonderful structure inside if the shell were whole.

The analogy here is too perfect to ignore. I am sitting with essentially a broken shell—my broken cochlear implant—and it's giving me an opportunity I wouldn't have chosen for myself, to experience a month without hearing. How many people can do that? Certainly not hearing people. Only someone in my unique situation, waiting for a replacement CI with the presumed good fortune to return to that world of sound at the end, could try such an "adventure." Just like Emily's broken shell, what new insights, experiences, and even wisdom will I find because it is broken?

What I've noticed most so far are the different reactions I've been getting. People with hearing loss—both hearing aid and cochlear implant users—understand completely the deprivation and panic that set in when I stopped hearing, and they immediately understand the stress, fear, and short temper. They know all too well how that feels.

The reactions of hearing people are somewhat different, though. They are supportive and shocked to hear the news, and they wish me well, but I can tell that hearing people took my hearing for granted. That was my persona—I could hear and they didn't really see a person who couldn't, even though intellectually they knew the implant was providing the sound. It's what I meant and referred to in that letter to the editor of the *New York Times*, referring to cochlear implants: "I doubt that hearing people will ever truly grasp the magnitude of this miracle." But now that it's failed—as they watch me move through the next few weeks in silence, see how this silence impacts our communication, and imagine more graphically just what it is like to walk in my shoes—they just might.

MARCH 21, 2008 Pre-Op Testing

I'm finding that dealing with the deafness and the isolation it brings is more stressful than I ever imagined. Trying to communicate all day long is so exhausting that I have to watch carefully how much I take on. Thoughts of doctors, appointments, surgery, recovery, activation—those will have to be dealt with one step at a time as well.

Yesterday was my pre-op testing and my appointment with my surgeon. I was very nervous about the testing and couldn't seem to calm myself down. It's probably just as I've described it—the stress from the lack of hearing and communication leaves no buffer zone to handle any additional stressor. And pre-op testing is stressful even if you can hear. I had given a lot of thought to how to handle the communication during these procedures, and decided that Ira would be my oral interpreter. I decided not to even try to lipread hospital personnel, as that would exhaust me both emotionally and physically. This is not my usual communication mode. Usually I proactively tell people I have a hearing loss. But this was different. With no hearing at all, there's no way that I could function there.

That was the plan and it essentially worked as I expected. The pre-op testing loomed very large in my mind as a hurdle to overcome: not just the communication aspect, but also all the pieces of it—so many pieces! Needles drawing blood; EKG leads being stuck on me; X-ray positioning; the interview with a physician's assistant using my oral interpreter husband; the consult with anesthesiology, again using my oral interpreter husband; and urine testing. For someone who is very private and quiet, this was a blur of assaults on every part of me—all done deaf.

And then the appointment with the surgeon, which went wonderfully well! This was the first time I had ever met Dr. Thomas Roland, and I was so relieved when he typed onto a computer screen so I didn't have to rely on lipreading. The calm that settled over me from that small gesture was palpable—no struggle to communicate.

When all the tasks of the day had been completed, I felt different. Some sort of transformation had taken place. This huge day's hurdle was over. I could now look optimistically forward to the future, something I hadn't really been able to grapple with before. Even though I was still dealing with the deafness, the slap of it—that intense sense of siege—had softened. My brain still hates it, but it is handling it.

That transformation is one of letting go—that I've turned the corner and am now someone who is waiting to get a new implant. It's a subtle shift in attitude—and getting through that pre-op testing seems to have been the catalyst. I'm still taking one day at a time, but my focus now is not really on how many days I've been without sound, but how many days until my surgery. I still get teary at times, but not overwhelmed with grief. Clearly, there has been a mourning process going on.

I've already learned some things while in this "broken shell" existence. Sometimes we are sent angels (or cherubs) when we least expect them. Sitting in that pre-op waiting room, there was a one-year-old baby who had one CI and was going to have a second one implanted the same day as mine, by Dr. Roland as well. His name is Nicholas; he has beautiful blue eyes and blond hair, and he loved Ira's sweater buttons. If I could tell Nicholas's family that he is in good hands and will be fine, I guess I should believe that message myself.

MARCH 23, 2008 The Secrets of the Broken CI World

I've been without sound for two weeks now and I think I've finally figured out the secrets of this Broken CI World. This is neither the hearing world nor the deaf world—it is My World. It is visible only to those who inhabit this special place—a CI user waiting to be reimplanted.

I've been dancing around the truths governing this world for days now. All the clues were there staring at me, but I had to live it for a while before it could make sense. Just like adjusting to the dim light of a darkened room, it has taken me two weeks to adjust to the rhythm of this world of silence.

This world is like no other, but it's my world now, and it's up to me to understand its basics. They are simple: I can't hear, I try my best, I sometimes cry—and if all goes according to plan, this world will come to an end with the insertion and activation of a new implant. It also doesn't hurt to keep one's sense of humor—if it can still be found.

It is vitally important to grasp the temporary nature of this world, so being optimistic is imperative! A positive outcome is highly probable, so it is counterproductive to dwell on low percentage possibilities, or waste time worrying about events that are unlikely to occur. With that as a given, this world has started to make sense.

Since this is a temporary world, the common coping skills and strategies used for hearing loss don't apply. For me, that means that my years of finely honed coping strategies must be tossed away. It is *not* helpful in this world to cling tenaciously to remaining active and involved in the hearing world. Those ingrained habits of using every possible assistive device, advocating for ones that aren't available, and making sure that if the world doesn't provide you with what you need, then you change the world: forget about that here in the Broken CI World. With no sound, I'm not equipped to function at all in the hearing world. Assistive devices—except for captioning—are useless, so trying to struggle where I just don't have the equipment or lipreading skills will end in exhaustion and frustration.

I couldn't have known this two weeks ago. Only after having some good experiences and some bad could I possibly know now what works and what doesn't. And living in this Broken CI World was the key.

Right after the devastating news at my audiologist appointment on March 10, effectively declaring that my CI was no longer functioning and that it had to be replaced, my husband and I went to a multiplex nearby that showed captioned movies. Why? Because we could. I could do captioned movies, and walking into that movie theater after such a blow, along with the silence, I felt human, that I could still do something "normal."

I also went to a captioned performance of *Spamalot* at the Kravis Center in West Palm Beach. I could do that, too. Even though I couldn't hear the music, the humor was right there on display for me to read—and I laughed out loud.

I gave a lot of thought to going to the Purim celebration at my temple. That's where they read the Megillah, the Book of Esther, with the tradition of dressing up in costumes and making a ruckus using groggers whenever the villain Haman's name is mentioned. I always loved wearing my best "diamond" tiara to the Megillah reading (Queen Arlene!). But the thought of silent groggers and not hearing Haman's name spoken at all, that was just too much for me to handle, so I stayed home.

And I also opted not to go to the anniversary service that my rabbi was conducting, even though Ira and I will be celebrating our thirty-eighth anniversary next week. I wanted to go, but Ira talked me out of it. He couldn't imagine me sitting there in silence, not hearing any of the music or the service—or the blessings. I thought it over and I had to agree, but it made me sad to have to forego this. It wasn't in my nature to give in to hearing loss, to withdraw instead of tenaciously remaining involved and active. But this is different—this is the Broken CI World, and I have no hearing whatsoever—and it is temporary.

Basically, whatever makes it easiest to get through the day, that's what is essential to do. If that means to withdraw, then that's the right course of action. To do otherwise results in exhaustion and frustration, and is simply not necessary. Using e-mail to connect with friends, or texting on the cell phone—that's the way most communication will be for now. Socializing in person with friends is definitely out—I wouldn't be able to hear them, and I don't want that kind of stress. For me, this goes so against my grain. It's a little hard to come to terms with what seems like retreat, but it's not retreat.

The other rule of this world: Save your strength and in-person contacts for those things that you must do. Whether it's job- or family-related, only do those things that would normally require hearing if they are absolutely essential.

This is not admitting defeat in this totally bizarre and unique world. Taking one day at a time, pampering yourself with things you can do without hearing—that will help make the days, if not pleasant, at least tolerable.

I'm not sure if this qualifies as the "wisdom" I was hoping to find, but it does feel like it. Looking back on the first two weeks, during which I was so stressed and distraught, with no buffer at all for additional stressors—it's good to know now that it doesn't have to be that way. And that once some semblance of acceptance is reached, it's possible to look ahead with some optimism and enthusiasm for the days when that precious hearing will return. Helen Keller said, "When one door of happiness closes, another opens; but often we look so long at the closed door that we do not see the one which has been opened for us."

That closed door was the wonderful hearing I had known for ten years with my old implant, and it's normal to mourn it. But now, with the will to move forward, it's possible to look at that new door that is now opening for me. The one with the new implant, the new technology, and the new possibilities in the world I long for so much—the hearing world.

MARCH 26, 2008 Adventures and Exhaustion

I've finally decided this is not a great adventure! The adventure part is right—there's no arguing that taking someone who has had ten years of vibrant and full hearing and plunging them into silence, rendering them unable to talk with fellow human beings, is an adventure. But it's not a *great* adventure, which implies a thrill worth trying. No—I would not recommend this to anyone!

The description that makes the most sense is one also attributed to Helen Keller, who undoubtedly was the expert on silent worlds. She said, "Life is either a daring adventure or nothing." And that does capture it. My brain knew there was something big about this experience that required summoning forth special energies that the hearing world never demanded. It had to respond to that challenge or fall away into oblivion. Enduring life in silence, shut off from communication with others—that is indeed a daring adventure.

I looked up *daring* and found *audacious bravery* as a synonym. Yes, that's what thriving—or surviving—requires in this silent world! In the beginning, I spoke about having a good attitude, but I know now that's a description for the hearing world. It's not merely a good attitude that's required to come through this ordeal with a positive outlook, but the will to make the most of it, and not become a muddle of defeat. So I pat myself on the back for discovering this trait I never knew I possessed—audacious bravery!

I've also written that navigating in this silent world is exhausting. I've used that word over and over, and it is still sitting flat on the page. Finally, this netherworld has produced the example I was seeking! My children visited me over the weekend, and I was thrilled that I could still lipread my daughter so well. Her last four years of high school coincided with the last four years before my cochlear implant, with my hearing so bad that she often had to act as my oral interpreter, interceding between teachers, friends, and the outside world. She complains now that she never got to rebel as a teenager, but acknowledges that it probably kept her out of trouble!

During our visit, I was able to chat pretty fluently with my children, lipreading with no sound, and enjoying the connection we could make despite the silence I was caught up in. We spent the afternoon together, and after they went home, I went up to my office. The next thing I knew, my husband was tapping me on the shoulder. I had fallen asleep while at work at my computer, sitting upright in my armless desk chair. I was lucky I hadn't keeled over and hit my head! Now *that* is exhausted!

Lipreading with no sound is insidious. It looks easy enough—the brain is obviously working overtime to scan visuals, vocabulary, context, grammar, logic, and topic to come up with the right words and responses. The physical exhaustion doesn't kick in until later. It's probably the stress of the give-and-take in real time with other human beings— constantly being pressed to respond on time, in synch, and right.

So audacious bravery meets total exhaustion. After seventeen days of this, yes, that sounds about right.

MARCH 27, 2008 Day Before Surgery

Tomorrow is the day that has been on my mind since all this began —March 28, the day of surgery. I have received many caring and loving messages, and they mean so much to me. I know myself by now and am seasoned enough to take things as they come. Maybe it's the maturity of age that makes one say, "Just do it and do not think too much about it." I talk a good talk, don't I?

Only a few days ago, I lamented my decision not to attend the anniversary service at my temple. I understood the rationale for the decision, but felt sad that "the silence" had won. Now I'm learning that the outcome of this decision is curiously full of wonder. I asked my rabbi to e-mail me the blessings he would have given in person, and this is what he wrote:

To you and Ira, we wish you mazel tov on the occasion of your wedding anniversary. On thirty-eight marvelous years, we wish you much joy and happiness. May your future days be blessed with the same love that you first shared under the chuppah—a love that was passed so clearly to your children, who fill their lives with the same caring, respect, and admiration that you have modeled for them. May all of the gifts that you have brought to each other over the years continue to overflow to touch the lives of your friends and family, our people Israel, and all of humanity. Amen.

I now have this beautiful blessing to cherish and keep. The last sentence is particularly meaningful to me, especially in light of my surgery tomorrow. I started losing my hearing soon after our wedding on March 29, 1970. I always felt that something good should come of my hearing loss, so I made advocacy a priority. As my hearing declined and I could no longer function, I received my cochlear implant in October 1997. It was as if I were being rescued so I could continue my work. It took a miracle, a true miracle, for this to happen.

Now, once again, it's time to move forward—with a new implant and a new direction. My grandmother always said, "We are all in God's hands." My grandmother was very wise.

Replacing the Cochlear Implant

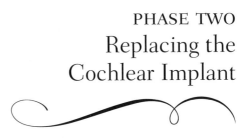

The day of my surgery finally arrived, a day I had been waiting so long for—in silence. Interestingly, my friend had had her cochlear implant surgery the previous month and put me in touch with Jody Gill, NYU Medical Center's Director of Language, Cultural, and Disability Services, the day before my surgery. Jody told me she could assist me in the operating room. I don't use sign language, but we would communicate by lipreading and note-writing. What a huge relief! From that moment on, I referred to Jody as my guardian angel! If you doubt this description, just imagine her holding my hand as they put me to sleep. She had also alerted the hospital staff that I was deaf, so they were attentive to my needs. I even had a whiteboard and marker to write notes if need be.

The surgery went well and was only about an hour long since there was no need to do any drilling. Thankfully, I had virtually no ill effects from the anesthesia, a very different outcome from my first CI surgery ten years before. The long consultation with the anesthesiologist prior to this surgery had paid off. I went home the next day, needing nothing more than Tylenol for pain.

The big hurdle was over, and now I had only four more days of silence to go. I was curious to see how the new state-of-the-art processor would differ from my old one. I figured others would want to know as well, so I continued writing . . .

APRIL 2, 2008 Activation Day—
I CAN HEAR AGAIN!

I hadn't realized how emotionally fragile I was getting to the activation appointment. I somehow couldn't summon up excitement for it. The emotional toll of these past few weeks without sound had been even more enormous than I thought—somewhat like being beaten up, pummeled. I think it was the surgery as the grand finale that sapped whatever emotional energy I had left, since I'm still healing up from that. I sort of limped to the finish line.

My first mapping session was actually uneventful and routine. My audiologist, Betsy, went through the various tones to determine my comfort levels. I didn't really know what volume levels were optimal, so I was conservative in my responses. We tried a few different settings to see what sounded best. We conversed briefly while she covered her mouth and I had no problem understanding her. Some sounds were a little strange, my husband's voice was too high, and mine had a slight boom to it—but I could understand everything without looking. It wasn't like starting from scratch. I was able to function well with the new processor right away.

I listened to some music and comedy CDs on the way home and my general impression was that I was catching more words than before, and even music was richer and more melodious. If I had to describe it, I would say that my brain didn't have to do as much of the work. It didn't have to push to imagine the music or work so hard to make the sounds into words. The voice of our car's GPS was exactly the same as before. The voice mail announcements on my husband's cell phone were extraordinarily clear—better than before. That's a first impression on just the half hour ride home. I could hear Ira in the car without looking, too.

I was watching television this evening and was surprised to hear that the voices were separate from the background music. I didn't have that kind of separation before. And my daughter called this evening, and I was able to speak to her on the phone with only a few repeats. I wouldn't hesitate to pick up the phone again.

My husband is delighted to have me responding to my name again, and all those other useful things hearing is good for. **We both realize that implanting the other ear is definitely something we plan to do within the next year.** Three reasons: First, I don't ever want to be without sound again if I can help it, so having a second ear as backup would preclude the situation I found myself in. Second, I really think the improved sound and music processing of this new processor is significant, and two sides would make it even more so. And finally, one never knows what the future holds, but if I'm physically able to withstand the surgery now, I'd like to do it now and not worry about what might be down the road.

I have another mapping appointment tomorrow and then another a week or so later, and then every few months on beyond that. This is not like my first CI activation ten years ago, though. The circumstances, mindset, emotions—this time I am bringing ten years of hearing to it. My reactions, perspectives, even who I am— they're all different now. Although I never would have chosen this particular path, I do think there is much to learn from it.

As far as the psychosocial aspects of this entire experience, things are starting to calm down. My husband, who really bore the brunt of this episode, is very relieved to have me back to talk to. He said that I was like a hair trigger, just as I've described—no buffer zone to cushion any extra stressors. I was on edge with everything. Now with the sound back, things are starting to relax and conversation can flow once again. It's much easier to readapt to living with sound than trying to function without it. That's an understatement if there ever was one!

We have a wedding to attend in two days, and it was against all odds a month ago that I was going to be able to hear at this event. It is a blessing to contemplate now.

APRIL 4, 2008 Reaping with Joy—
The Wedding

I was really looking forward to this wedding, particularly since just three weeks ago, it seemed like an impossible dream to be hearing again by April 4. To get through evaluations, pre-ops, surgery, and activation in so short a period of time, especially since we had been in Florida and had to get back to New Jersey, was almost too much to imagine. But taking things one day at a time, with a lot of support from friends and family, got me there!

The folks at NYU scheduled my activation just five days after the surgery. Their priority was to get me back to hearing ASAP, and they did! My sutures are still behind my ear and are coming out in a few days. My scalp still feels a bit numb, which I expected, but let me tell you, it's a whole lot nicer recuperating while being able to hear! There's not that much swelling, so the magnet is sticking, and that's an important consideration as well.

I've been doing very well with this new processor, but with a mere two days' experience, I was content to be able to go to this wedding *not* in total silence. The processor still has a high-pitched tilt and I've been told to expect that as my brain starts shifting things around in the adaptation process. But I can hear with it—even the telephone is good—so I knew I'd be okay at this wedding.

Driving there, we put some news and music on the radio, figuring it would give my brain as much practice as possible. One never knows what this brain can do with even a few minutes of practice. It's amazed me before! The wedding and reception were being held at Battery Gardens, a restaurant at the tip of Manhattan overlooking the harbor, Ellis Island, and the Statue of Liberty.

Once we got there, I found that the acoustics of the place were not to my advantage—all hard surfaces and high ceilings. The background music plus the sound of a lot of people conversing just registered as a blur, but I could actually hear voices through that blur and didn't find myself struggling. Bear in mind that this could also be the cumulative effect of having to lipread for almost a month without sound, but I would have felt that tug if I were struggling. I was hearing enough speech sounds through the noise not to fret.

What I was really looking forward to was the ceremony, so I took a seat on the aisle, close to the chuppah and in view of the rabbi. When the rabbi began the ceremony, I could understand her voice pretty well, especially when I was in view of her face, but I was working at it. The real surprise—actually shock and awe—came when she began chanting the first prayer, the *Shehecheyanu*. For me, with a processor so new that my brain was still hearing things relatively high-pitched, the voice of this rabbi/cantor was a gift beyond imagination. She was a coloratura soprano! When she opened her mouth, I couldn't believe what I was hearing—a beautiful stream of melodic tones, warbling gracefully with vibrato. I hadn't heard vibrato like that in decades! I had been able to hear beautiful singing with my old processor, but nothing as magnificent as this.

It was totally unexpected. I'd only had this processor two days! But the bigger impact was actually in the meaning of that particular prayer. My understanding of the *Shehecheyanu* prayer is that it is said at certain holidays and life cycle events, but it can also be a way to offer thanks for new, unusual, or exciting experiences. The translation is: "Blessed are You, Lord, our God, sovereign of the universe, who has kept us alive, sustained us, and enabled us to reach this season."

What a wonderful proclamation welcoming me back to the world of sound! Tears welled up in my eyes as I sat in utter awe, trying to absorb what was happening. Just a few weeks ago, I was shedding tears of grief and frustration, and now I was crying with joy! And this morning, my husband kept smiling at me, calling me his "miracle girl."

"Those who sow with tears shall reap with joy." —Psalm 126:5

APRIL 10, 2008 From Silence to Sound—One Week

Those twenty-four days of silence are actually starting to become "the past." The experience is starting to mellow a bit. Time is starting to heal that wound. I know that many people were hoping that my time without sound would go by quickly. I never really shared that hope—only that I would have the strength to get through it, and maybe even learn from it. In many respects I have. For all the talk about the awe, wonder, and miracle of hearing again, whatever emotions I had before are tenfold now. I guess there's nothing that makes one treasure something even more than having it taken away for a significant period of time.

I visited Dr. Roland again to remove the sutures. This was the first time I had actually heard his voice. He didn't do my first CI surgery ten years ago, so the first time we met was three weeks ago when I was already without sound. In that shroud of silence, we could barely communicate with each other; writing notes was essential. Now that I could hear his voice and actively converse, it was as if we were meeting for the first time. I asked him about implanting my other ear. He told me I should wait six months to give my ear a chance to adapt to my new processor. That made sense to me, and also added to my resolve to pursue "going bilateral."

I've been driving with the radio and CDs on, trying to compare the sound of my new processor to the old one. I'm able to hear dialogue through background music a lot better. Before, when I put the news on the radio, I could never understand the "headlines" because of the background music. Now I seem to have a fighting chance. And music sounds like music—none of that "electronic mush" that took me months to adapt to with my old processor. There's also no doubt that there's more separation of voices and instruments. For example, the Simon and Garfunkel song "Scarborough Fair" has a very complicated, interwoven harmony. With my old processor, I'd never heard the intricacy of those inner voices that I'm hearing now. When watching television, I'm picking up a lot of speech without looking. What really took me by surprise was hearing a voiceover in a commercial that had background music. That's something I never would have heard with my old processor. And, in general, I'm hearing better in noise. It just seems easier.

In a store today, I heard piped-in music with astonishing clarity. With my old processor, I remember being so impressed to hear music at all in the stores. Who knew, right? Today, the music was so clear and distinct, it was a little scary. I hadn't really expected to have one of those I-landed-on-a-new-planet type of revelations, but I'm using this new super-sophisticated technology, so it makes sense that I'd notice some striking differences.

For a situation I never would have planned on my own, I'm finding myself looking forward to enjoying the newness of it all. I'm incredibly relieved, though, that the big stuff—silence and surgery—is behind me.

APRIL 12, 2008 Compare and Contrast

Now I'm starting to have a bit of fun with this new processor. (Fun wasn't in my vocabulary two weeks ago!) Most of the aftereffects of the surgery have worn off, and I'm getting my stamina back and renewing my activities—still sore and healing, though.

I can say that the sound I'm getting now is almost what I would consider "normal"—not the tinselly high-pitched sounds I started with. My brain seems to have gotten that accomplished. I know from my "new processor" experience ten years ago that the more listening practice my brain gets, the faster it learns and adapts. It's like feeding the scent to the bloodhounds—it runs with it.

Listening to that Simon and Garfunkel CD, for example, I noticed more complex harmonies than before. But the sound of the music was still a little thin at first. Two days later, the same CD sounded richer and more robust. My brain has done this before—it's tentative listening to something the first time, then "gets it" the next time. Knowing this, the best strategy is to do a lot of listening, so it can get past all those "first times."

I've also noticed that this processor preserves the background noise, so you're aware of it, but it doesn't drown out speech or music. This came up as I was listening to an announcement on a classical music station for an upcoming string quartet concert at Carnegie Hall. There was a string quartet playing in the background and I not only heard the announcement, I could also hear the string quartet accurately as well. The same thing happened with an announcement for a piano recital, with a piano playing in the background. I had never been able to hear an announcement through background music; it would always blend together. This was novel to me—hearing both separately and accurately like that. I really would like to know how this processor knows how to *do* that—sort out the music from the voice-over—especially since they're both using the same frequencies!

I also seem to be able to hear people from a greater distance. I was in an informal social situation where a group of women was seated around a room, speaking one at a time. I could hear their voices across the room—not perfectly, but enough to be able to follow. I don't think I could have functioned in that environment with the old processor, not from that distance.

I'm noting these listening experiences because they are significant changes from my old processor. I feel as though I'm being showered with rosebuds that are blossoming. As the sounds of my new processor gain greater richness, depth, and clarity, a floral shower is the perfect metaphor for beauty and rebirth, so vastly different from the ugly silence I endured so recently.

APRIL 28, 2008 Some New Tricks

I just learned that this processor can do another trick the older one couldn't—hear all around me. I was sitting on the left side of a bus, with my implanted ear next to the window. There was the incessant drone of the bus engine, ventilation system, and road noise, so I was a little surprised to have my brain alerting me to someone speaking nearby. That's exactly what it felt like, as if it were tapping me on the shoulder saying, "Pay attention, Arlene—I hear someone talking!" I looked around, and on the other side of the aisle, one row back, were two young men talking to each other. I couldn't hear exactly what they were saying, but almost—I still needed to look at them. *Hmmm . . .* This processor was pulling in speech from that distance on my *other* side over all that bus noise? This is definitely better than I expected!

I've continued to play CDs in my car, and one easy listening recording with jazzy arrangements of old standards has become my favorite. I discovered that I could identify two of the songs, "I Left My Heart in San Francisco" and "Mack the Knife" through the bluesy piano, trumpet, and saxophone arrangement. They were *not* playing the melody in the high frequencies—it was embedded in the harmonies. I was a little surprised because with my old processor, I usually had to be told what the song was before I could recognize and appreciate it. Being able to hear the individual voices through the harmonies allowed me to identify the embedded melodies. I was in new territory here—identifying songs for myself!

I played this entire jazz CD while driving with my husband, and he mentioned this was the first time we'd ever listened to a purely musical CD in the car together. He's convinced that this behavioral shift is because of my new processor and its better rendition of music. I agree.

And I can't believe the BIRDS! Evidently, this processor has more "reach," so it is able to field even distant sounds clearly. My outdoor walks are now *filled* with symphonies of chirping birds, from trees near and far. I was able to hear birds with my old processor, but never like this!

MAY 18, 2008 Doing "Better"— Gold, Silver, Bronze

Adapting to a cochlear implant is always about doing *better*, yet what does that really mean? It's easiest to understand by dividing hearing into three categories:

GOLD—normal hearing, being able to hear words without visual cues, and comprehending them instantaneously

SILVER—being able to understand words without visual cues, but requiring mental effort to process their meaning

BRONZE—needing visual cues to comprehend speech with the proportion of each varying. As speech comprehension diminishes, reliance on visual cues increases.

Speech comprehension is also impacted by noise and distance, so we find ourselves in four basic situations: quiet/near, quiet/far, noisy/near, noisy/far. CI users do best in quiet/near situations—with many people functioning at either Silver or Gold levels of hearing. But it's when the environment gets more challenging, at greater distances and noise levels, that assessing how well we're functioning becomes more difficult. Using these Gold/Silver/Bronze categories provides a benchmark to measure progress.

It seems that all my functioning has shifted for the better with this new processor. Listening situations that had been Silver are now Gold, and some listening situations that had been Bronze (needing visual input) are now Silver (no lipreading required). The shift is mainly due to this new processor being able to handle distance and noise much better than the old one. Moving toward the Gold and Silver categories and out of the Bronze, relying less and less on visual cues, is at the very heart of doing *better*.

This week, I saw people at an arts access committee meeting that I hadn't attended since getting my new processor. These meetings provided real-time captioning and I could always function acceptably well by listening and glancing at the captioning when needed. As soon as this meeting began, I knew I was doing *better*. That shift in functioning I just mentioned—going from Bronze to Silver and from Silver to Gold—that's exactly what was happening here. I could hear several people at this meeting without having to look at them. The processor was bringing in their voices in a way that was almost like using an assistive listening device! If I missed something, I simply glanced at the captioning screen. At the end of the meeting, the captioner said that my new processor was going to put her out of business! She was watching me and noted how little I was using the captioning.

As I was heading out the door, I heard someone speaking to me from behind. I turned around and saw one of my colleagues about ten feet behind me. I was just about to ask him to repeat what he said when my brain informed me that I already knew what he said! With one second's worth of reflection, I realized that I had, indeed, heard him tell me, "Have a safe trip home!" I had never been able to hear from behind like that before, especially so unexpectedly. It's a clear illustration of what it means to do *better*!

MAY 20, 2008 Moving Toward Bilateral

I attended a presentation at NYU Medical Center on bilateral cochlear implants. The timing of this workshop was impeccable—I had now recovered from my surgery and was ready to move forward with my plans to go bilateral. I was still a little tentative and figured that more information would give me the confidence to proceed. This was the perfect opportunity. The entire NYU CI Team was there—doctors *and* audiologists!

Unfortunately, there were no assistive listening devices at this session and the person who was supposed to provide the real-time captioning had canceled at the last minute, so I was on my own. Again, my new processor pulled in the speech sounds, allowing me to hear loudly enough and clearly enough, with visual cues, to function.

I learned that speech comprehension actually improves with bilateral CIs, as does directionality and functioning in noise. And a new study had just come out showing a significant increase in the quality of life for people using bilateral CIs.

This session was just the push I needed to start the process of going bilateral. I arranged to have the three-month evaluation for my current CI also serve as the evaluation for the bilateral implantation qualification process. Once that was completed, I could obtain my insurance pre-certification and then schedule the surgery—moving one step closer!

MAY 31, 2008 Patience and Piano

I haven't mentioned it, but I've been playing the piano again. Music, in general, has been wonderful. I did well with music before, but with this new processor, most instruments and harmonies are better—even listening to the piano. But, *playing* the piano is something else again.

I had taken piano lessons as a child and into my teens, playing in various concerts and recitals. The pieces I played were all memorized. As my hearing declined to severe and profound levels, I stopped playing. After all these decades, two pieces—a Schumann *Arabesque* and a Chopin *Nocturne*—still remained "in my fingers." What's different this time around from my first CI ten years ago is pitch and harmony. With the old CI, the piano sound was "warpy" and my brain had to work to supply the pitches. Too many keys sounded the same or similar, the chords would run into one another —my brain was trying too hard to make the music sound right. I know now that it just didn't have the tools to do so. But now, with this new processor, it does!

The piano still sounds warpy, but the notes have more definite pitch. My brain doesn't have to guess at what I'm playing, and that has made all the difference in my inclination to continue. I haven't reported on this because there wasn't much to report—I was playing, it still sounded warpy, but I wanted to continue. Now, after eight weeks, the piano is sounding a little less warpy, and the harmonies are starting to sound—dare I say it—beautiful. Both of these pieces have a very definite melody, and I'm finding myself really pouring my heart into the music because it now has pitch. My brain is singing along, not having to manufacture the notes. I'm not getting sidetracked as before, trying to make it music. It *is* music.

There's more to it than that, though. We tend to concentrate so much on speech, which is our primary goal with our CIs, that the other textures of life's tapestry are often relegated to the background. But for those of us who once had normal hearing, our lives are intertwined with the sounds we once heard. That Schumann *Arabesque* was the theme song of a program on WQXR, the classical radio station my father always listened to when I was growing up. He was a high school instrumental music teacher—just like in the film *Mr. Holland's Opus*—and music was his life. When I added this Schumann piece to my repertoire, he was thrilled, and always loved when I played it. Of course, as my hearing diminished, I stopped playing that and everything else. He passed away in 1997, and we wanted to inscribe something meaningful on his gravestone to reflect his love of music. We chose the first two measures of that Schumann *Arabesque*.

It's an interesting turn of events, playing the piano once again, although it's not at all like when I was sixteen. Back then, I could play and hear the notes perfectly. Now, the tone sounds a little warpy, and the pitch is hardly perfect. But there's no doubt that when I sit down at the keyboard, I bring an intense depth of emotion and maturity to the music that no teenager could possibly possess.

JUNE 8, 2008 TV as Therapy

Did you ever feel that you were being manipulated by events, that you were making choices, but that the path was already determined? My travel plans for getting to the Hearing Loss Association of America (HLAA) convention in Reno were just like that. I've been actively involved with HLAA for many years, and now, as president of the New Jersey state association, I looked forward to attending this convention.

There were no direct flights to Reno from any of the New York City area airports—just flights with time-consuming layovers. The only itinerary that made any sense was flying JetBlue from JFK to San Francisco, renting a car, and sightseeing our way to Reno. We've always flown JetBlue to Florida, preferring it because of its seatback TVs. My husband loves them, but I usually prefer doing Sudoku and crossword puzzles, and maybe glancing at a cooking show occasionally.

Here's the scenario: I had just had a mapping session two days before, we had a six-hour flight to San Francisco on a plane that had seatback uncaptioned TV screens, and we had to bring our own headphones since JetBlue was no longer giving them out. As we took off, I put on my headphones and started flipping through the TV channels. I finally had control of my own clicker! I dabbled through the History Channel, the Travel Channel (learning how to do a decent hula dance), then on to the news, hearing some cabin announcements from the captain as well.

It was slowly dawning on me that I was hearing and understanding everything, and also that this felt strangely similar to the many hours of listening to books on tape that I had done ten years ago as auditory therapy. But this was different because this was not just dialogue—it also had background music and noise, and I wasn't missing a beat or a word. I wasn't really focused on this, though. My mind was intent on writing up the experiences I've just related in the previous episode. I was doing that by hand, in ink, on a yellow legal pad.

Out of a six-hour flight, my guess is that I was watching and listening to TV for about four hours, and since the sound was going directly into my processor via the headphones, that would most certainly qualify as auditory therapy. I did absolutely *no* Sudoku puzzles and not a single crossword—my brain was otherwise engaged!

As we walked to retrieve our luggage, Ira said he noticed that I had been watching, and watching, and watching the TV, so he surmised that I was understanding the dialogue. I'm sure that using my own better-quality headphones had something to do with this success, but there's no doubt that being able to extract speech from background noise was the primary factor—something I'd always had difficulty with using the old processor.

Recapping the situation: Because of the quirks of the airlines' schedules from New York to Reno, as well as headphone policy changes, I ended up flying JetBlue using my own good-quality headphones to effectively give me four hours of auditory therapy of a type (TV listening) I never would have thought to do on my own or had the opportunity to try for that length of time. Excellent "planning," Arlene!

JUNE 12, 2008 B and B and Yosemite

Planning our itinerary to Reno for the HLAA convention, we had decided to stay at a bed-and-breakfast inn just outside the western entrance to Yosemite National Park. We had never been to this park before and looked forward to spending the next two days there. It was an informed decision to choose a B and B, not something I took lightly. Staying at a B and B is a decidedly interpersonal experience—effectively being welcomed into someone's home and being treated like long-lost relatives. It is very social, interacting with the host innkeepers when arriving and also at the trademark breakfasts. Most people with normal hearing probably don't realize that to truly enjoy a B and B experience, you have be able to hear! In my pre-CI days, it was essentially solitary confinement at the breakfast table—something I decided was not fun and came to avoid, even though I loved the Victorian architecture and furnishings typical of this type of accommodation. With my old CI, I could hear and function well enough to enjoy the B and B experience, so that was put back into our repertoire of lodging choices. And so we came to stay at the Yosemite Rose B and B in Groveland, California, for two nights.

Sure enough, upon ringing the front doorbell, we were greeted by Katherine, the hostess and innkeeper, who would take us on a tour of the house, show us our room, and settle our accounts. Ira immediately spied a Yamaha baby grand piano in the front parlor and nudged me to sit down and play while he took care of the paperwork with Katherine. I was a little surprised to have my piano-playing skills displayed so soon. I had only started playing again a few weeks ago! But I was a good sport, knowing that I had practiced enough to play at least a little in public. I sat down and played some Chopin, and later learned that Ira was telling Katherine my entire CI-user-turned-pianist story. Without missing a beat, we got the rest of the house tour, learned that I was free to play the piano until 9:30 PM, got our luggage up to our room, and were off to our first peek at Yosemite! We didn't get back to the inn until 10 PM, though—too late to tickle the piano keys.

The next morning, breakfast was on a lovely, sun-drenched screened porch, hosted by Don, Katherine's husband. This is what makes B and Bs unique—the innkeepers treat you as guests in their house, which means chatting over breakfast. There were two other couples, each at separate tables, which meant we were pretty spread out on that porch. Even so, I was doing fine fielding all the voices. Not surprisingly, the topic of conversation turned to hearing—it's always like that. Don immediately asked me about the feedback he was getting from his hearing aid. That one was easy—the tubing on his hearing aid was old and brittle and needed to be replaced. Another guest then owned up to the fact that he had poor hearing in one ear and wasn't in a rush to do anything about it. I ended up counseling about hearing aids and assistive listening devices all through breakfast, actually enjoying the challenge. Personally, I was delighted to be following all this conversation, parrying the questions from all sides!

We again headed into the park, spending all day there, but this time returning by 9 PM. Ira looked at the piano, looked at the time, and asked me if I could play. It would just be him as the audience. I'm still a little perplexed at his enthusiasm about my piano playing. At first, I thought it was pride in having his wife sit down and play, and that's certainly what happened when I played for Katherine. But since we were alone now, there had to be a different motivation, and I think I understand it. Ira's bride in 1970 could play the piano— and hear. We got our baby grand in 1973 when I could still hear well enough to play. With my CI, I have been hearing again for more than ten years, but the piano playing must have been missing from Ira's life as well as my own. We are so often focused on our own hearing, on our own functioning, and on concentrating on our own progress that we forget that our hearing impacts those closest to us as well. Hearing me play brought back a piece of our lives from a more innocent time, and along with it the joy we associated with it. So I played—Chopin and Schumann—in our private little concert at the foothills of Yosemite.

The next morning at breakfast, everyone wanted to know if I was the one who had played the piano the evening before! Oh my!

Evidently I did have an audience after all—tucked away in their bedrooms, but listening to the concert below! I had made my CI piano debut and didn't even know it. I didn't even have a chance to get nervous!

As we were getting ready to leave the B and B, Don followed me to the door and thanked me for giving him so much information about hearing aids the day before. He and Katherine also asked me about getting a CI for his ninety-one-year-old mother. (It seems that everyone I meet always has elderly parents who can't hear well.) I told them their best bet was probably a small one-on-one amplification device. With that last piece of advice, we all hugged at the door, they walked us out to the car, and we departed one last time for Yosemite.

As we motored over the mountain roads, Ira said to take it all in because it was unlikely we'd ever pass this way again. Those words sounded so familiar, and I thought immediately of the following quotation, something I'd always taken to heart:

> I expect to pass through this world but once. Any good thing, therefore, that I can do or any kindness I can show to any fellow creature, let me do it now. Let me not defer nor neglect it, for I shall not pass this way again.
> —Stephen Grellet, 1773–1855,
> French-born Quaker Minister

These words were so true of this Yosemite B and B experience—driving up out of nowhere, touching our hosts' lives, and being embraced by their warm hugs in return.

We spent the rest of the day touring Yosemite, and as we made our way over the mountains to Reno, Ira asked me what I enjoyed most. His favorite part was touring the Mariposa Grove, with the giant sequoia trees. We had ridden a tram into the grove and everyone had been given an FM receiver and headphones they could tune to the language of their choice. I enjoyed that, too, since I didn't miss a word. That was in contrast to the bus tour we had taken the day before to Glacier Point, the magnificent vista overlooking Yosemite Valley. In that tour, I couldn't understand enough of the driver's speech to be helpful, but I knew not to try to lipread him because then I'd miss the vistas—a lesson I had learned the hard way many years ago!

The answer to "my favorite" was really quite easy. It was lunch in the dining room of the historic Ahwahnee Hotel in Yosemite. It wasn't just the food or the surroundings—it was the total experience. We had wanted to have dinner at this hotel's landmark restaurant, but when we asked Karen at the reservation desk, there were no suitable times available. Karen seemed very nice, though, so we chatted a bit, learned what her favorite menu item was (trout *almondine*), and I asked her if it was possible to have lunch there instead. She said, "Of course!" and told us to come back in twenty minutes when she'd have a special table ready for us. We did just as she instructed, and when we arrived, she escorted us like VIPs down the entire length of the magnificent 1920s grand rustic restaurant and seated us in front of the two-story floor-to-ceiling window that overlooked the majestic rock cliff and waterfall scenery. I immediately turned to Karen and told her that I felt like the Queen of England! She didn't bat an eyelash, replying that the Queen had actually sat at the next table over on her last visit! For someone who has a collection of tiaras and Queen Elizabeth dolls back home in New Jersey, this was definitely what I would consider the proper way to go camping in Yosemite!

I can't say for sure how different this B and B and Yosemite experience might have been with my old CI. Certainly, I wouldn't have played the piano there, I might not have been able to follow the breakfast conversation as well, and I might not have had as much confidence to start chatting with Karen at the Ahwahnee restaurant reservation desk. I mention all this now at the ten-week mark to give you an idea, once again, of how my new processor can work in unexpected ways to make life more enriching and enjoyable. And I also can't help but think, *Let me not defer nor neglect it, for I shall not pass this way again.*

JULY 6, 2008 Three-month Real-life Evaluation

I decided to do my own three-month evaluation and not wait for the "official" one next week, with all the words and sentences to repeat. Those tests are valuable to clinicians, perhaps, but the real evaluation is out in the real world, with real listening situations. The Fourth of July weekend gave me ample opportunity to assess my functioning, so here's my real-life three-month evaluation report of my new processor.

We attended the Fourth of July celebration in Ridgewood, New Jersey—a bedroom community of New York City that on July 4 seems much farther away than its half hour commute. This is "Smalltown, USA," whose July 4 tradition spans almost a hundred years, including a folksy parade that features local marching bands, fire engines, politicians, and school floats, followed in the evening by a band shell concert and fireworks. With that as backdrop, here's how my new processor fared:

MUSIC: Only one band actually ended up playing music as it passed by our spot along the parade route. But after hearing just a few bars, I instantly blurted out, "That's the 'Washington Post March!'" And my husband verified that I was right! With the old processor, I might have recognized that it was a march, maybe even a Sousa march, but I'd usually have to be told what music it was first, and then fit that information into what I was hearing. But with this processor, I could play Name That Tune!

CASUAL HEARING: This category is how I would describe being receptive to spoken language even if you were not alerted to the fact that someone was speaking to you. This is a new category needed for this processor—I couldn't really do this very well with the old processor. In this case, we were milling about the sidewalk table where they were selling and taking tickets for the band shell concert and fireworks, when I distinctly heard from behind, "Do you need an extra ticket?" I immediately turned around and said, "Yes, I do," and a man just handed me a ticket. It all happened so fast, I'm still amazed!

SPEECH DISCRIMINATION: We were seated in front of the band shell, a good distance from the loudspeakers, awaiting the start of the concert. There was an introductory speech being given, along with a welcome by Ridgewood's mayor. I heard it and understood it through the loudspeakers even before I could locate who was actually doing the speaking onstage. We were too far away for lipreading, so this was without any visual cues. I know I couldn't have understood this well with my old processor, but my husband may be getting used to this because he didn't even try to tell me what they were saying. He only commented that the speeches were mercifully short.

LOUD SOUND PROCESSING: The fireworks provided the test to see how this processor handled overly loud sounds. The volume wasn't too loud or too soft—it was *just right*! During the grand finale barrage, the booms were too loud for my unimplanted ear, the one that can only hear explosions, yet the volume was still *just right* for my new processor.

We continued our "Fourth" celebration on the fifth at a social gathering with friends and family. That provided more test results.

HEARING IN NOISE: I was at a table for eight with lots of other conversational noise all around, and was in there functioning. I definitely needed to look, but I was usually just one repeat away from understanding if I needed it.

VOICE MODULATION: I had ample opportunity to talk with my cousin, an audiologist who knows me, my hearing, and my voice very well. She told me that my voice was the best it's ever been—that it is deeper, has more resonance, and has no nasality at all.

DEMEANOR: This is a new category, too, prompted by how this processor has affected my behavior. I was told by one of my friends who hadn't seen me since getting this processor that I look more relaxed. I know that I'm having a much easier time understanding her (she has an accent), so I must be doing less *processing* than in the past. This dovetails with the relaxed demeanor others have mentioned during the meetings I've been attending.

Unlike the official three-month evaluation with word and sentence lists and percentage scores, there is no way to assign a numerical value to this real-life evaluation. I'm content just to call it *better*.

JULY 10, 2008 Official Three-month CI and Bilateral Evaluation

July 9 had been circled on my calendar for a long time now. It was the date of my three-month evaluation for this new processor. I never liked evaluations—never liked being scored, ranked, or rated—and that goes back to school exams, term papers, and employment evaluations. Soundproof booths added even more emotional baggage. Those cubicles were all bad news for the twenty-five years I was losing my hearing. I'm no newcomer to CI evaluations, either, and realize that I'm not the one being tested—it's the CI processor that is. That sort of reasoning was fine for my first processor ten years ago. But that was then. This is now.

This isn't just any processor. This is the processor for which I essentially waited ten years of CI usage and twenty-four days of silence. This isn't some detached piece of electronics anymore, as it felt like it was ten years ago. My CI is a part of me now. I know what it's like when it doesn't work. I'm a long-term CI user and I have a lot of emotions invested in a device that connects me to the world.

With that as background, I was downright nervous coming into this evaluation. I had put a lot of effort into adapting to my new processor—listening to all sorts of sounds, speech, and environments.

I knew I was doing well with it, but I still had to "perform" with it. I really shouldn't have been nervous, though, because this wasn't just a three-month evaluation—it was also going to be my bilateral CI evaluation. The bilateral evaluation was testing the unimplanted ear to see if it heard poorly enough to qualify for a CI. I had already done this back in 1997 when qualifying for my first CI then. My hearing surely hadn't gotten any better over the years (I had just spent a month in silence!), so I knew before anyone did anything that I would qualify for the CI in that ear. No need to be nervous about that. Failing that test was a desirable outcome!

The tests would involve my CI alone and in combination with my other ear, which was being equipped with a hearing aid for this session. With that variation added to the stew, along with a completely new battery of tests geared to assess functionality in noise, this turned out to be more about the *other ear* than I had anticipated.

Two years ago, I had tried putting a hearing aid in that ear, and although we came up with an aid that might have worked, I discovered that after a two-hour fitting session, I wasn't hearing as well with my CI on the phone. I pulled the plug on that project immediately! So walking into this evaluation, red flags went up when I realized that my brain was going to be coping with my CI and a hearing aid. I warned my audiologist that my brain would start favoring the hearing-aided ear, skewing the test results; but we had no choice but to plow ahead with the tests—pure tones, single syllable words, sentences, and then the grand finale—noise.

I noticed that the usual volume level on my CI sounded particularly strong that day, and I was almost tempted to turn it down, but I didn't. We started with the other ear, which was now fitted with a hearing aid. It still has some low frequency hearing, but zero speech discrimination. Actually, it seemed worse than when it was tested ten years ago—there *are* gradations of zero. When it was time for my CI-alone testing, the volume of my CI now seemed too low. Uh-oh—my brain had started to morph already, but what could we do but continue?

Results? On the sentences, I got 100 percent when using both the CI and the hearing aid. With the CI alone, I got 96 percent.

With my old processor, I always got 100 percent on sentences. So from an unenlightened point of view, it would seem that I did better with my new CI in combination with a hearing aid. But the reality, according to me, is that using the hearing aid degraded my functioning—temporarily—with my CI. The whole issue is moot, really—because the functioning is still excellent. The single syllable word functioning was 80 percent with the CI alone, compared to 72–74 percent with the old processor in years past. So there was improvement there. How much the hearing aid impacted my functioning on that test is unknown. Even without asterisks of explanation, I'm still doing better on single syllable words with this new processor than with the previous one.

The noise tests were very elaborate, geared to test functioning in each ear alone and then together—presenting sentences with noise in front, on the left, and on the right. This was the first time I'd ever had this type of evaluation, so I can't compare it to my old processor, but my audiologist said I did very well in noise with my new CI.

The verdict on my other ear is that although it still has some low frequency hearing, it is not giving me any benefit, and I would likely do better having a CI in that ear. So the bottom line of this evaluation is that the right ear is definitely a CI candidate! One other curious result of this bilateral testing: My brain was giving me good vibes on hearing with two ears. It was subtle, but when I had to go back to hearing with just the CI, it just didn't seem as natural. Part of that is probably the low frequency hearing that's lacking in the CI. But Mother Nature gave us two ears, so it makes sense that brains are wired to want them both to be functional.

How did this official three-month evaluation compare to my own real-life assessment of my new processor? It was good as far as it went—and I know that these tests have to be limited and uniform, but it was lacking in a few key areas that are also predictors of functioning. It only used a man's voice, so there were no high-pitched chipmunks in that cubicle. The speech source was only three feet away, so there was no indication of how I'd hear at a distance. And, of course, we didn't play Name That Tune—an understandable omission since we were assessing speech proficiency. From the discrimination and noise tests, I could see why I was able to respond to someone talking to me from behind—extracting the speech sound from noise at close proximity, ie, *casual hearing*. But the test couldn't predict how I would do in more trying situations where speech is farther than three feet away—and that comes up a lot in real life, and is something I know this new processor does better than the old one.

On paper, I do look as though I've fully adapted to this processor, and my audiologist told me as much, but I know that's not the case yet. But now that the three-month evaluation is over, I'm ready to relax and enjoy the benefits of this processor, let the sounds flow over me, and note any "CI moments" as they may occur. I need to do this. It's time to smile and turn the page to a new chapter.

JULY 20, 2008 Wake-up Calls

I thought that after my three-month evaluation, I would just smile and move on. I thought that I had adapted enough to this processor not to have to concentrate so hard. I thought using a headpiece with a weaker magnet could alleviate the minor discomfort I was experiencing at the magnet site. That had happened before and had solved the problem right away. Alas, I thought wrong, wrong, and wrong.

After my three-month evaluation, the irritation I was feeling at the magnet site that day got worse, not better. I was starting to feel sensations at the top of my head, the incision site had started to ache, and even my outer ear hurt. It wasn't really bad enough to call pain, but it was enough to take some Tylenol to alleviate it.

But then I realized that the scalp numbness that I had been experiencing since the surgery was starting to abate. It felt as if my scalp were "coming alive" again. That surprised me because after my surgery ten years ago, it took over a year for that numbness to go away. I should have been happy, but now it seemed that as the numbness was lifting, it was revealing pains, discomforts, and sensations that I hadn't been aware of before. I should mention that I'm very sensitive to pain and discomfort—very. What most people would not even be aware of or find bothersome, I often find intolerable. I watch people laying on a beach basking in the sun and wonder how they can actually enjoy that when, for me, it feels like my body is being torched doing the exact same thing. My brain can detect and get upset at having even a grain of sand between my toes. I sometimes wonder if this qualifies me as a bona fide princess! It can have its benefits, but in cases like this CI magnet (or being a canary in the mine), hypersensitivity is definitely a negative.

Now it was starting to make sense that the magnet had probably been too tight for a while, but the sensation was being shrouded by the numbness. I had gotten no advance warning, so by now, the discomfort was considerable, at least to me. I started to get a little panicky, wondering if I would have to cope with pain just to be able to hear. I kept the processor off for several hours in the morning, and I put some folded-up tissue under the magnet, to make the pull weaker. I figured this would help let the site heal. My husband took a look and saw nothing unusual there—no redness or swelling. So it was literally all in my head, but I still had to deal with it.

It wasn't getting better, though, and that night I woke up at 4 AM, in what I've come to call a *monster attack*—all the fears and thoughts of the day gaining on my brain until it's forced to wake me up in a flood of tears. I've had this happen before, but not in a very long time. I used to wake up like this almost every morning in the years before getting my CI, in a panic about how I would get through the next day. I learned how to deal with it and handle it rationally, in spite of the hysterics and tears.

The first thing I do is turn on the light because laying in darkness without hearing is stressful even under the best of circumstances. Once the light is on, the talk begins and the fears start flowing. My husband is quite understanding of this and knows to give me time to talk and calm down. I couldn't imagine what the solution to this situation would be—I already had no extra magnets in my headpiece. Would I have to endure pain and discomfort just to hear—forever? At 4 AM, probabilities don't mean much. Worst case scenarios prevail. When I had calmed down enough, the lights went off, and I went back to sleep.

In the morning, I e-mailed my audiologist, who arranged to have a lighter headpiece shipped overnight to me. And the next morning, it was right there on my doorstep. I also e-mailed my surgeon, describing what was happening, and he responded that this was all within the normal range of recovery. I e-mailed with people in an online support group, and they all said this goes away. The new headpiece is lighter and it does connect, just barely enough to stay on my head, but it's working and I can hear with it. I also changed to the smaller, lighter battery, which I discovered lasts over twelve hours, so that's helped as well. The uncomfortable sensations are still there, but are calming down—and with it, my anxiety level.

I'm still a little perplexed, though, about the 4 AM monster attack with its tearful hysterics. It's been years since I've had an episode like that. In this instance, I was clearly overwhelmed—I had been through my CI failing, being plunged into silence for twenty-four days, then pre-op fears, the surgery itself, anticipation of the activation with hopes of being returned to hearing, and then the adaptation process, culminating in the three-month evaluation—and now fears that I'd have to endure pain just to hear. I had every right to cry!

I had always thought these 4 AM anxiety episodes were a sign of weakness, that I was a puddle of mush in the face of adversity. But seeing the facts surrounding this episode and thinking back to the previous ones, I think the veil of tears is a rallying call, a summoning of strength to go forward "tomorrow" and deal with the problems. It's useful to take a look at what actually did happen on all those tomorrows: The problems were fought through and dealt with, not always easily, but usually with tenacity. Instead of thinking of this process as going from crisis to crisis or problem to problem, perhaps what we're really looking at here is going from strength to strength.

"They go from strength to strength, every one of them . . ."
—Psalm 84:7

JULY 26, 2008 The Persistence of Memory

Thankfully, my new, lighter headpiece has been working out better for me, and the troubling sensations and discomfort have been getting progressively better. I'm almost to the point where I don't notice having anything on my head, and I do hope that continues! I'm now ready to try, once again, to relax and enjoy the benefits of this processor. I really would like to take a time-out from intense listening analysis and just let the sounds flow over me, letting my brain do whatever it feels like doing. As a seasoned CI user, I don't feel compelled right now to push hard to practice listening to recorded books or other audiotherapy strategies. I'm a little tired and would just like to coast a bit, allowing my brain to engage in free association, taking in sounds and sights and doing with them whatever it likes.

So now—once more with feeling—I am smiling and moving on. Without even paying much attention to it, I've noticed that there are rarely any "chipmunky" voices anymore. Some voices on the radio and television are still problematic, but, as per my "moving on" plan, they'll be what they'll be for now, and I just don't want to think about it!

One voice that had that chipmunky quality was my exercise instructor, Janet. Once a week, I attend a class that concentrates on weight-bearing exercises and working all the muscle groups. Per my "princess" constitution, don't even ask me what weight strength I work out with. Suffice it to say, it's enough for me! Janet talks nonstop during the class, not only giving instructions, but also chatting interactively with us about anyone and anything. She now sounds almost normal, with only tinges of that chipmunk quality to her voice.

Every so often, Janet introduces some new approaches to old routines. At the last session, we were seated on the mats with our legs somewhat contorted, and she told us to lift one leg up a few inches. I did it, but not easily. "My brain is not happy about this, Janet!" I called out. She looked back at me quizzically. "Your brain?" Uh-oh. I just realized that I was now in the real world, the hearing world, and no longer in my enchanted CI realm where brains rule. Hearing people don't usually refer to their brains in the third person! Well, it's their loss that they don't understand that every-thing that happens to them is at the pleasure of their brains! So I explained that their brains were giving them feedback during all the exercise maneuvers in this class! Whether it was the balance exer-cises ("Hang in there, we can do this!") or which weights to work out with ("You expect me to lift *how* many pounds? Okay, we'll give it a try."), or those new routines ("You have to be kidding—we weren't meant to do this!"). To me, it seemed quite routine to see everything in those terms. I'm still not quite sure that I convinced Janet of that, however.

In the same spirit of just basking in life's sights and sounds, I've also continued to play the piano, but without the pressures of tonal-ity, pitch, or technique. Instead of stressing myself to learn anything new, I've been playing the same two pieces again and again—just altering the tempo and phrasing. I was particularly intrigued by how I could vary that Chopin *Nocturne* each time. I decided to slow down the tempo, which made it sound much more mournful, almost like a serenade—a love song. As I was playing it this way, my brain informed me, "You know, that's exactly the way you played it the day Kennedy was shot!"

WHAT!!!!???

And then I began to recall the events of that day. Everyone of a certain age remembers exactly where they were and what they were doing on November 22, 1963. I remember first hearing the broadcast announcing the shots at 11 AM, and then at 1 PM, the pro-nouncement that the president was dead. I recall coming home from school at 3 PM. My house was empty, I was alone, and I didn't really know what to do or how to handle the enormous emotions I was confronting. I sat down at the piano and played—yes—that Chopin *Nocturne*, though not at the normal tempo. I played it slower, to make it sound more mournful, almost like a serenade—a love song. I remember the thought process—the perfect emotional outlet of a young teenage girl who had just experienced the loss of her dashing young president. I never played it that way again—until yesterday.

That was almost forty-five years ago. How did my brain get to this deeply embedded past? I've been playing that Chopin piece for weeks now, with no rustling of that memory. But this time, I had allowed my brain to roam free—no pressure to work on anything. And as with any free association process, as the theory goes, sooner or later it will stumble across a crucial memory. And so it was here, with the enhanced sound of this processor, resurrecting a bittersweet memory—an auditory memory—stored away a long time ago.

AUGUST 4, 2008 The Ultimate Computer

We were out to dinner with friends this week, and I was thinking how wonderful it was to hear across the table, even with some moderate background noise, and still be able to follow a three-way conversation. The table discussion turned to politics, and I found myself not even thinking about hearing, but thoroughly engaged in the issues instead.

And then, just like last week, my brain informed me, "You know, this sounds exactly like the conversation we had four years ago— your friend's voice, the same intonation, the same phrasing, the same preachy arguments—just the specifics are a little different. And you were convinced he was totally wrong then, too!"

Oh my—it seems that my brain is now routinely doing memory searches based on sound. This is the second time in a week! And I have to admit that this recollection was exactly right—again! During that last conversation four years ago, I held my tongue. This time around, following the conversation was so easy (plus finding that history was repeating itself so irritating), I immediately became embroiled in the heat of the argument. What I learned from this empowering experience is that the age-old adage about not discussing religion or politics in polite company is still probably the best advice!

I remain intrigued, though, about my brain using sound to retrieve memories. The brain is, after all, the ultimate computer, its search engine far more complex than Google or Yahoo. It even has the capability to store and retrieve memories based on scents and sounds! But—and this is a big *but*—only if those capabilities are *enabled*.

I did have sound in my life, except for the twenty years when I was losing my hearing, so my brain is searchable for sound—even CI sound. The improved speech and music capabilities of this processor have evidently enhanced my ability to retrieve memories—short- and long-term—and presumably to create them as well. A new dimension has been added to my life!

I acknowledged just a few weeks ago that "my new processor can work in unexpected ways to make life more enriching and enjoyable," but this memory capability is *so* unexpected and *such* an enrichment, I can't seem to get it out of my mind! The ultimate irony.

AUGUST 14, 2008 Behaving Myself

I'm now past the four-month mark, and I'm feeling a little smug that I've gotten through some thorny patches of chipmunks, hoarseness, head soreness, and general adaptation blues. I know I'm hearing *better*, and what's intriguing to me, now that I've had some interesting listening experiences with this processor, is that *better* isn't just about hearing. It's also about behavior.

Ten years ago, when describing what it meant to do *better*, I only thought in terms of hearing. I knew that being able to hear again would enable me to function in the hearing world, something I couldn't do before. At that time, the contrast between hearing and not was so stark, that's all that really mattered. It took several months to adapt to the realities of hearing again, changing from a person who shunned human interaction into one who welcomed it.

Over the years, I became an expert at knowing how I would function in a variety of situations, and it shaped the activities I chose to do and also those I avoided. After ten years, I had gotten that act together pretty well. I knew that I needed captioning for television, movies, and theater to greater and lesser extents depending on the programming. I also knew how well I could expect to function in a restaurant, around a dining room table, at meetings, and in casual conversations. My hearing shaped my experiences, and my experiences shaped my behavior.

Now my world has been shaken up with a new processor whose improved technology and capabilities are again impacting my behavior. I'm particularly intrigued that, with this processor, my brain doesn't have to work as hard to hear. It's starting to dawn on me that if my brain is not working as hard to hear, then what is it freed up to do? THINK!

Yes—think! In that political argument I had with my friend around a dinner table just a few days ago, I heard his voice right away. I didn't have to work to understand it. That freed my brain to remember a similar conversation four years before, and then to start ranting and raving about politics. Even I was surprised at the fierceness and passion that was pouring from my mouth! This seems to be similar to the way baseball players put donut weights on their baseball bats during practice so they can swing faster and stronger when they're batting during a game. That's just what happened with that political argument. My brain has been so used to working to hear (my baseball bat donut) that when that burden was lifted, it was free to launch a political diatribe of home run proportions! (I also learned that I'd better rein in that passion a little bit in the future.)

Something similar happened this past weekend. We were going to see an outdoor performance of *Hair* in Central Park. Before the performance, we were casually discussing the show around the dinner table, and one of my friends mentioned that the casting call had been restricted to people under the age of thirty. I immediately shot back that I could have played almost two people! I said it *so fast* that everyone stared at me—and then laughed. Evidently, my brain was accustomed to having to think to hear at a table conversation like that (my baseball bat donut again), but with this processor doing better in casual conversation, my brain was freed up to launch one-liners at breakneck speed.

I thought about that Chopin piano experience where I retrieved a forty-five-year-old memory from the day of Kennedy's assassination. This processor was able to deliver better pitch, so I enjoyed playing the piano again. But delivering better pitch also meant that my brain didn't have to work to manufacture its own (that baseball bat donut again), leaving it free to launch a memory retrieval expedition four decades deep!

Will this phenomenon start to slow down as I get used to this? I'm not sure. What seems to be happening is that, at least in these instances, my brain was freed up to retrieve information and make connections. Interestingly, those are also the skills that are needed to do crossword puzzles—and I do lots of crossword puzzles. My crossword skills have definitely improved over the years, and I do them faster, too. Now this seems relevant to my hearing in an interesting way. Once my brain was freed up to do something other than process hearing, it did what it thought it had been trained to do all these years—retrieve information and make connections.

As a reality check to all these positive events, though, I still encounter negative situations as well. Some noisy party situations—notably those in small Manhattan apartments—still give me a hard time. I also find that the acoustics of a space continue to have a big impact on how I function, but that's nothing new. Some phone situations are also more difficult than others, with voice quality and connections varying. I'm still figuring this out, deciding whether mapping changes or just more time adapting will smooth away these problems. But they do make me a little hesitant the next time if I've had a difficult experience.

This is all part of the learning curve, with subtle shifts in my general behavior emerging as a result. It's impacting my responses, my demeanor, my body language, my memories, my sense of humor —in essence, revealing more about myself than I expected.

AUGUST 24, 2008 Arts and Crafts

Florida in August doesn't conjure up the most enticing image, yet that's where I've been for the past several days. Heat and humidity plus impending hurricanes don't sound idyllic, so what could possibly have drawn me to this part of the country in the summer? The answer is simple: one of my favorite events, an arts access conference that was being held this year at the Broward Center in Fort

Lauderdale. I've been attending these conferences for the past six years because their agenda dovetailed with my agenda. Access to the arts has been one facet of hearing loss advocacy that I am particularly passionate about, with captioned live theater being one of my proudest advocacy accomplishments.

Some of the "hearing angels" that helped make captioned live theater a reality in New Jersey and on Broadway are also founders of this annual conference, along with others just like them. After attending one conference, I was hooked. It was also a treat to attend a mainstream conference that graciously provided full communication access for me (assistive listening devices and captioning) at all workshops, receptions, and entertainment. The experience has always been a little slice of heaven.

As I entered the Broward Center, I saw the person who had done the captioning for *Spamalot* at the Kravis Center last March—the one I attended in silence, but laughed out loud at because I didn't miss a word. I'm not usually the huggy, emotional type, but I found myself wrapping my arms around him as if I were some long lost space traveler arriving back on Earth! That was the only emotional association with my device failure that I experienced returning to Florida. With everything else, I just picked up where I had left off—or so I thought.

During the conference, one person commented that I seemed calmer, not as tough or intense; another person alluded to my smiling demeanor. I've always been quite outspoken at these conferences and I didn't think calm and smiling were what defined my persona, so I did a quick mental checklist to see what, if anything, might have changed.

Hmmm . . . I really thought I was as outspoken and pleasantly tenacious as always, not saying anything particularly different or less emphatic than before. But then I remembered the other meetings I've attended recently and the comments people had made about my relaxed demeanor. I know that I'm hearing better and am more connected to my surroundings, not working as hard to hear, responding more quickly in casual hearing situations—all skills that are particularly helpful at conferences like this one. Now I'm wondering what my more relaxed body language and facial expressions are conveying! I would love to think I was exuding an air of confidence and authority!

And, as usual, someone approached me at the end of the conference, in tears because she was losing her hearing. She had heard all my comments regarding the needs of people with hearing loss, she had admired how assertive I was about my own needs, and she told me she was now inspired to face her own hearing loss and do something about it. This episode, however, had a strange twist. This woman had been a sign language interpreter for the past twenty-five years! I guess that lays to rest all the ill-informed comments people have made to me over the years, asking why I didn't just learn sign language instead of getting a cochlear implant. Here was a woman who knew exactly the impact of using sign language instead of hearing to function in the world at large. Her tears when confronting her own moderate hearing loss said it all.

That was a fitting finish to this conference, learning once again that hearing loss is far more complex than we ever imagine—and also discovering that in the real world, hearing is also about relating to people.

AUGUST 25, 2008 The Sand and the Sea

I couldn't leave Florida without taking a walk on the beach, something I enjoy immensely. The last time I did this was back in March when the waves and the wind were silent. This time, the glorious sound track was back! I thought of that beautiful prayer sung in my temple, "Eli, Eli"—even more meaningful today than when I heard the sounds of the ocean with my first CI ten years ago.

> Eli, Eli—oh Lord, my God,
> I pray that these things never end,
> The sand and the sea,
> The rush of the water,
> The crash of the heavens,
> The prayer of the heart.

The sand and the sea,
The rush of the water,
The crash of the heavens,
The prayer of the heart.

I had always thought this was an ancient prayer. Just recently, however, I learned that it was originally a poem written by a young Hungarian woman, Hannah Senesh, who had settled in Palestine in the late 1930s. During the war, she was part of an underground rescue effort, one of twenty-four people airlifted into Yugoslavia in an attempt to assist the besieged Hungarian Jewish population. She was discovered, tortured, and killed at the age of twenty-three. In a notebook she had left behind in Palestine was her poem, "Eli, Eli." It was subsequently set to music and has become part of the traditional liturgy in many services, sung in both Hebrew and English.

Twenty-three was the age I got my first hearing aid. Hannah Senesh's life journey was ending at the point where my life journey was beginning. Knowing this history gives yet another dimension to this experience. And adding still more, I just received the pre-certification insurance approval for my bilateral surgery, scheduled for September. That means there's a very good possibility that I will be listening to the ocean with both ears on my next walk on the beach—God willing.

PHASE THREE Bilateral Cochlear Implants

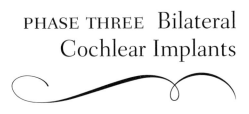

AUGUST 31, 2008 Thinking Bilateral

My bilateral surgery date is only ten days away and I have to admit that I'm getting excited and nervous at the same time. I think they call this *approach-avoidance* in Psychology 101: You truly want something, but it has other qualities that make you want to avoid it. That pretty much describes the situation of ardently wanting to hear with two ears, yet having to endure surgery to get there.

Helen Keller has said, "Life is a daring adventure or nothing." Being plunged into twenty-four days of silence when my CI stopped working was definitely a daring adventure. Going through the reimplant surgery process was a daring adventure. Exploring the world of sound with a new processor for the past five months has been a daring adventure. When I decided to go bilateral, I knew that the surgery and activation would be yet another daring adventure, but a necessary one if I wanted the chance to hear optimally.

Now, with the surgery date so close, I'm starting to imagine what hearing with two ears might be like. There's no doubt that receiving my medical insurance pre-certification approval has fed this bilateral thought process. It was all hypothetical until that *yes* came through a few days ago. Now reality is starting to set in. I'm surprised that I'm even allowing myself to get excited about hearing bilaterally yet—I'm usually too much of a worrier. But I can't seem to help it. I haven't had two ears working together in over thirty years!

As if on cue, "thinking bilateral" cropped up yesterday. Ira and I were at an outdoor antique show in Connecticut, an activity we've always enjoyed because, even when my hearing was declining, it was something we could do together. Until I got my CI, though, I couldn't chat with the dealers, something I thoroughly enjoy doing now. But hearing or not, I've always loved walking through open fields searching for treasures. My trademark lately has been to wear a wide-brimmed sunhat that is color-coordinated with my outfit. Yesterday was apple green. As I was walking along, Ira informed me that one of the dealers had just complimented me on my hat. I hadn't heard the dealer talking. He was about twelve feet away on my right side—my unimplanted side. Interestingly, Ira said that if I had CIs in both ears, I would have heard the compliment. *Hmmm*—yes, that's probably true. And, *hmmm*—it seems that my husband is now "thinking bilateral," too!

We finished the antique show early and discovered an impressive clock museum nearby. Connecticut was once known for its many fine clockmakers—Seth Thomas, Sessions, Waterbury—and this museum had rooms full of clocks of all types. At 2:55, we found ourselves surrounded by grandfather clocks. I was really looking forward to hearing the clock chimes with my new CI processor. At the stroke of 3:00, the clock symphony began—chimes, dings, bongs, and bells—all enchanting and melodious. But I had no idea which clock was making which sound! I have no directionality with my one CI, and I immediately thought how nice it would be to hear with two ears, and know which clocks were chiming.

It almost sounds trivial the way I've just described it—wondering what it's like to hear a room full of chiming clocks with two ears. But when else could I possibly indulge myself in this kind of serendipitous speculation, except when awaiting my next "daring adventure"—bilateral surgery.

SEPTEMBER 7, 2008 Out of the Comfort Zone

The days are going by one by one, and it's now less than three days until my CI surgery. I've just gotten through the pre-op testing, and being able to hear this time made it a lot easier than it was back in March when I couldn't. I got the same nurse again and, amazingly, she remembered me because I was so upset last time. She seemed so nice now. Everyone was so nice—something that had totally eluded me when I couldn't hear.

I'm using all my wits to keep my stress level down, but the nerves are running at full throttle. I'm not even sure why my body is tensing up so much this time around. I've decided to write about this because if I don't, I might create the impression that I either have nerves of steel or that it's simple to go through the surgery and recovery process.

Intellectually, my mind says, "Just do it, and stop thinking so much!" Good advice. I'm wondering, *why* am I thinking so much? Because the choice has been totally mine, electing to do elective surgery. Last March, when I had to replace a broken internal component, there was no question that I had to go through the revision surgery to get my hearing back. This time, that's not the case.

I have chosen to pursue the long-term benefit of hearing bilaterally, knowing full well it entails another surgery and recovery. I knew I'd eventually have to confront these difficult days. I'm still comfortable with the decision—wanting to go bilateral—for many reasons. But I knew I would be pushing myself out of my comfort zone to do it—and now I'm here, confronting the realities of that decision.

I had a discussion with my son about this concept—deliberately pushing yourself out of your comfort zone to attain long-term improvements. He had just given a talk on this subject, relating how he had confronted his fear of talking to his college professors by tackling that problem head-on, volunteering to be the student/ faculty liaison when he reached graduate school. He knew that taking himself out of his comfort zone would result in the personal growth he was seeking.

Looking back, I can cite several examples of when I've made similar decisions, but none is quite as simple or basic as the time I lost my first baby tooth, at age six. This almost sounds too silly to mention, but even after all these years, I remember it vividly. I still sucked my thumb at the time, and my older sister told me that my teeth would grow in crooked if I didn't stop. Talk about putting yourself out of your comfort zone—this has to be the epitome of the concept! Poor little Arlie—what to do? I did it! I remember making the decision—consciously and rationally deciding that my future smile was worth removing my thumb from my mouth forever! All you need to do is look at the cover of my first book, *Hear Again*, to know that I got it right!

And here I am again, sitting smack outside my comfort zone, wanting and waiting to hear the world through two ears. The idea of smiling on another book cover sounds very appealing right now, too.

SEPTEMBER 16, 2008 Arlene's Electrifying Bilateral Cochlear Implant Surgery Episode

It's about time I described what happened on September 10, the day of my bilateral cochlear implant surgery. I had arranged to have Jody Gill, the hospital's Director of Language, Cultural, and Disability Services, assist me through this hospital stay once again. Thank goodness for Jody, NYU's guardian angel of patients with hearing loss! She's a certified sign language interpreter, but for my purposes, I needed her as my ombudsman. Just as hospitals have specialists to monitor all sorts of patient needs, Jody was there to address my communication needs. Last March, I knew I had to have her with me, essentially functioning as my communications assistant since I had no hearing at all. This time, however, I was a little hesitant to ask for her assistance because I now had my hearing back. But I quickly realized that having a CI in a hospital brought its own set of needs, so I again requested her assistance during my stay.

Ira was with me as we arrived at the hospital's intake desk. I had just gone through this surgery process last March, so the surroundings and procedures were very familiar to me. One big difference was immediately apparent this time, though—I could hear! This wasn't going to be another surgical silent movie! The sound track was on!

We went through the sign-in process and I could hear the intake person and answer for myself. Then we met Jody in the pre-op suites. That's where you meet with everyone involved with the surgery and do all the last-minute protocols before the main event. This time, I had a chance to chat with Jody in a very relaxed manner. It was almost as if we were meeting for the first time. That's what deafness does to your personality and personal interactions—it's as if you aren't really there if you can't hear. Any conversation concentrates on *just the facts, ma'am*. There's no energy or inclination left for pleasantries or chit-chat—it's all business. But now, able to hear, I was engaged in some heavy conversations with Jody about how to get the word out about what she does and how she can help other hospital patients with hearing loss—and we would need to think in terms of not just this hospital, but other hospitals as well. What a difference being able to hear makes. I was alive again!

We were told that the surgery had been delayed a bit, and we would need to wait. I figured I'd go for a bathroom break, and as I opened the door, the anesthesiologist was standing there in front of me, about to knock. I recognized him immediately as the one from my last surgery. I joked that now that I had my cochlear implant, I could hear him knocking before he actually did so—the superpowers of being bionic! This immediately set the tone—that the person he had seen last time was but a shell of the one standing before him, able to hear, communicate, and be herself.

We sat down together and went through the details of the anesthesia, focusing on what had worked last time to avoid that dreaded hyperactivity side effect. I was visited by several other nurses and hospital personnel as well, including my surgeon, who marked my right earlobe with an X. When the operating room nurse came in, I recognized her from the last surgery, and she recognized me. This was starting to feel like a reunion, except this time I could hear everyone! I arranged with Jody to leave my CI processor on in the OR until I was put under. Then she would take it off, put it in a case, hold on to it, and put it back on me in the recovery room. That was the plan.

I walked with Jody and the OR nurse down the hallway. They don't wheel you in. It's sort of civilized and actually less scary that way. When I got into the OR, everyone had surgical masks on. We all know those masks, which make lipreading impossible and strike fear and dread in the hearts of people with hearing loss. But not me, not this time around. We had prepared for this. Jody kept her mask on this time, too, and she talked near my CI processor to make sure I could hear her.

As they were prepping the IV line on my right hand, the anesthesiologist was doing something on my left side, and he said to me, "We're attacking from both sides!" I heard him say it, and I immediately shot back, "I better cover my left flank!" Oh my goodness! Arlene's brain, hearing with her new processor, can fire one-liner retorts in an operating room filled with people with surgical masks on?! That surprised even me! This was not the OR experience I had ever known, that's for sure! Anesthesiologists had never joked with me before! People treat you differently when they know you can hear them.

Jody then told me they were ready to put me under. She held my hand, and I started to feel a little woozy, and that's the last I remember. I assume she took off my CI processor and held it because the next thing I knew, I was waking up in the recovery room, and I could hear. Jody had put my processor back, inserting the headpiece under the bandage that was now wrapped around my head. Ira was now standing by my bed, fervently hoping that I wouldn't have any problems with the anesthesia. This surgery had been longer than the one in March, so I had more drugs in my system, but I was still okay, and relieved.

I was resting comfortably, but wanted to get cozier, so I started pulling the sheets closer around me. Ira knows that I like to submerge myself under the covers, so he watched as I pulled the sheets up to my chin, then over my mouth, then under my nose. But then I stopped cold and exclaimed, "Oh no! This is a really bad place to pull a sheet over your head!" And with that, we both burst out laughing! Yes, being able to hear in the recovery room was definitely a different experience. It let me stay connected to everything around me, and then some!

We were also very grateful. Here I was, a deaf person lying in a hospital recovery room from surgery to restore hearing in my other ear, all the while being able to hear, talk, and laugh. We felt truly blessed.

I don't remember much else, but Ira told me that I was answering all the nurses, no matter where they were around my bed. He also said that I was being very funny. He also noticed that the more morphine they were giving me, the less funny I was becoming.

They wheeled me up to my room, and unlike other CI centers that send patients home the same day, I was kept overnight. Jody had sent detailed instructions to the nursing staff, and they placed a sign over my bed that said I was hard of hearing. I watched the clock all night, even though I tried to nod off, but I didn't sleep a wink. In the morning, the residents came in to check on me and removed my bandage. Jody came back to assist when the nurses gave me my discharge instructions. I didn't really need her, but it was still a good idea to have her there. She was rephrasing the instructions, just to make sure that I understood. Having just gone through surgery, anesthesia, and a sleepless night, one doesn't argue about getting some extra support.

Ira was delayed coming to pick me up. It was September 11, and the traffic into the city was extra heavy because of the memorial ceremonies that day. But he finally got there and we returned home. I'm not one of those people who runs marathons the day after surgery. Far from it! I was able to send a few e-mails out from my BlackBerry, telling people I had survived and was on the mend. But "just rest" was the order of the day, and the week ahead.

I didn't need any of the heavy-duty painkillers, finding that Tylenol was sufficient. For the first few days, I had a loud hooting sound emanating from my ear, but I found that if I put my CI on my other ear, the tinnitus went away. After a few days, that hooting stopped. I didn't have any dizziness.

And so ends the tale of my Bilateral Cochlear Implant Surgery. It was definitely more rigorous than the replacement surgery last March, but it was easier in one respect: I could hear through the entire experience. And that, as they say, is priceless.

SEPTEMBER 18, 2008 Bilaterally Enabled

It's been one week since my CI surgery, and I'm still a little sore, a little tired, and not quite myself. But the realization is slowly sinking in that I did it! All those months of waiting and wondering and nervousness—they're over! I'm on the other side of this surgery, and my world is very different now. Even though I haven't heard anything yet with my "new" ear, that's just a matter of time and electronics. I am now wired for sound in two ears—bilaterally enabled! That was the goal—to be able to hear with two ears—and I'm there!

What I wrote just ten days ago, that I was "outside my comfort zone, wanting and waiting to hear the world through two ears," wasn't quite accurate. The goal wasn't really to hear the world through two ears—it was only TO BE ABLE to do that! It was the raw capability of being able to hear that I was seeking, not the delightful sounds I might hear or the increased benefit I might derive. I wanted the reassuring knowledge that I now had backup, that if one side couldn't hear—for whatever reason—I would no longer be plunged into silence. *That* is what drove me out of my comfort zone to pursue this bilateral CI.

It's hard to believe that as recently as last February, I was very happy to hear with one ear and a ten-year-old processor. That was all very comfortable, and I would have been fine to exist like that indefinitely. People had been asking me if I was considering going bilateral, and my answer was always "NO!" But when my processor stopped working and I could no longer hear, my world changed dramatically, and so did my priorities.

Not only did I worry about not having a backup ear in case my processor ever stopped working again, but the possibility also existed that at some point in the future, I might not be healthy enough to sustain a replacement surgery. It was clear to me: The status quo was no longer acceptable.

And now it's done! Accomplished! Fait accompli! Goal met! The feeling is amazing—watching the plans develop and then come to fruition. And yet as I sit here writing this, it brings to mind a similar episode in my life where the status quo also was not going to be good enough. I'm surprised I hadn't thought of this before, as it extends far beyond the concept of comfort zones. Maybe intense experiences give rise to intense memories.

It was over thirty years ago that I was expecting my first child. The pregnancy was normal, but the labor and delivery were very difficult. The fetus had turned in the womb, and they needed me to be able to feel the contractions to help push the baby out while they used forceps to assist. They let the anesthetic wear off to do this. Don't even ask about the pain—I don't want to describe it. As the baby was being pulled out, they gave me some sort of gas to ease the pain, and I remember thinking that I was dying and wondering if I should tell them, but that they probably already knew. And then it was over. I wasn't dying, but I did have an eight-pound healthy baby boy—Michael. He was pretty beaten up and had a fractured clavicle, but otherwise, he was perfect! Needless to say, however, I wasn't in a rush to do that again.

Three years passed, and I still wasn't ready to face another pregnancy. But then I had to have an ovary removed, and my whole world was shaken up. I had no backup anymore, and the possibility also loomed that I might not be able to have more children. The status quo was no longer an acceptable option. Ten months later, Michael's sister, Emily, was born—with no extraordinary pain, heroics, or trauma. I remember being on cloud nine just reflecting on the chain of events, with its "bundle of joy" outcome.

I'm not surprised that I'm reminded of this now. The situations are so similar—facing the total loss of hearing or the capacity to have children, because there was no longer any backup, and then deciding that the status quo was no longer acceptable and finally facing down my fears to do something about it.

These were not small decisions, yet I think people might relate to the desire to have more children as the more courageous or *important* one. That's why I want to reiterate here and now that I doubt anyone who has never experienced twenty-four days of silence, after being immersed in a world full of sound, can possibly understand the intense emotion of *never* wanting that to happen again. At least now I know I've done all I can to mitigate that possibility.

With two more weeks to go before activating my new ear, I guess I'll indulge myself in some romantic thoughts of what it might be like to hear bilaterally again. The last time I could hear with two ears, Michael was just a baby.

OCTOBER 1, 2008 Waiting

I'm sitting here in limbo—the surgery is over, I'm pretty much recuperated, and I'm awaiting my activation tomorrow. Pretty boring here, but that's not necessarily a bad thing! I've taken some very good advice and rested—a lot—trying to recoup my energy. I had been trying to get back to normal, but I was still getting sleepy and tired, so I backtracked a bit and slowed down, napping and resting more than I might have. Definitely a good idea!

I haven't ventured out much into the real world, so from what I can tell, the world still sounds pretty much the way it did before the surgery. The right ear that I just implanted wasn't much use to me. It was only good for two things: hearing explosions in the movies and hearing the string bass on my jazz CD. I knew that implanting that ear, though, would likely destroy whatever hearing it had left. I wasn't really concerned about the movie explosions, but I was a little apprehensive about finding out if the string bass was now gone forever.

No sense keeping you in suspense: the string bass is gone. I drove to the post office a few days ago, and very tentatively put my car's stereo on—loud—wondering what that jazz CD was going to sound like. I had actually practiced this moment several times in the months prior to the surgery, plugging up my right ear with my finger just to see how things would sound. So it wasn't a surprise that my jazz CD lacked that grounding string bass accompaniment, but that's not the end of the story!

Evidently my brain realized that it wasn't getting the bass input it had come to expect, so it embarked on a *correction*. For the next two days, my CI sounded too loud and I had to turn down the volume on the processor—a sure sign that my brain was working on something. When things calmed down again, I noticed that my hearing had changed. Very interesting. I went back to the jazz CD again, and there was still no string bass, but the music sounded more mellow and *bassier*. Virtual jazz? My piano doesn't seem to have been affected by any of this, probably because the volume isn't loud enough to make a difference. But I am getting the feeling that my brain has transferred some bassier sounds over to the CI side, now that my right ear is no longer supplying them. Nothing scientific here—and certainly nothing major—but there has been a slight shift. All this is going to be moot anyway when they wake up my right ear with the CI stimulation tomorrow! But it did give my brain something to play with while waiting.

The timing of this waiting period and activation is also rather curious. These past two days, I was sitting in temple, attending Rosh Hashanah services. This was the first time attending a service since my surgeries. It had dawned on me a while ago, when I made my surgery and activation appointments, that if all went according to plan, I would be hearing with one ear on Rosh Hashanah, but with two ears on Yom Kippur, which is the following week. What curiously impeccable timing—the end of one era and the beginning of another.

As the Rosh Hashanah service began, I realized immediately that with this new processor, the music sounded better without an assistive listening device—the cantor, the choir, the organ, the electronic keyboard—all of it! Listening directly made the sound richer, fuller, more nuanced. I even preferred following the service in the prayer book listening that way—I could hear the page numbers being announced and could follow the text without a problem. The only time I used the system was during the rabbi's sermon.

Without getting into the details of religious belief, basically Rosh Hashanah centers on looking at the past year, evaluating it, and planning to improve in the new year. It also focuses on the premise that there is a plan set down for the new year, sealed at the final blowing of the shofar on Yom Kippur.

I have my own personal feelings about beliefs and faith, something borne of my own experiences and pragmatism. To reflect on the past year, it's hard to imagine that there wasn't an elaborate plan in place. In essence, I began the year as an older CI user who shunned any thought of another CI surgery or going bilateral, and am ending it as a bilateral CI user with two state-of-the-art implants. To accomplish this feat—including providing me with strong moral support along the way (my angels!)—I had experienced a device failure, endured a month of silence, gone through replacement CI surgery, adapted to a new CI processor, and had a second CI surgery, all the while being encouraged to chronicle these experiences. If I had to guess, the year-long mission seems to have been to eventually produce a book that shows: a) how to cope with a sudden hearing loss or device failure, b) how new CI processors differ from old ones, and c) what it's like to adapt to bilateral hearing. It's not a path I would have chosen for myself, but we don't always get to choose.

Tomorrow, the day of my activation, is a total unknown. There are so many variables, and only one brain to figure them out. The best I can do is what I've done these past few months—stay focused, stay positive, and hope the angels are standing by.

OCTOBER 2, 2008 Bilateral Activation!

Today was Activation Day. I had been looking forward to this day for a long time—and boy, was I nervous! This was the third time having a CI activated, and one would think it would get easier, but that is definitely not the case! Each of my activations brought with them a unique set of emotional baggage, fears, and expectations.

The first one, eleven years ago, was one of frightened awe—not really believing that I would be able to hear again, and even thinking that I might not even remember *how* to hear!

The second one, after the replacement surgery this past April, was as nerve-racking as it comes. I was totally deaf going into that one, desperately wanting to hear again, and petrified at the (improbable) possibility that it might not work.

This time, intellectually, I realized that I shouldn't be nervous. After all, I could already hear with my existing processor. My brain, however, doesn't always operate on that calm, intellectual level! Hearing—anything to do with hearing—evokes emotional responses in me. So that's how I was—the closer we got to activation time, the more nervous I became.

My appointment was at 2:30 at NYU's CI Center, and Ira and I left ample time to get into the city. We've evidently started a tradition here, that Ira only attends activations, not mappings. He's there not only to observe the process, but to lend moral support and a shoulder (and handkerchief) if need be!

As we drove into the city, Ira put on the CD of a recorded book, a biography of Albert Einstein. I started to listen along with him, but the subject matter and language was very heavy, full of scientific terminology, and as the road noise got louder, it was getting to be an effort to listen. I didn't want to wear myself out, so I just tuned it all out, preferring to work on a crossword puzzle instead.

We had no traffic, so we were very early. I had no inclination to go for coffee or walk around the neighborhood. All I wanted to do was sit in the waiting room and wait! As we got closer to the NYU building that houses the CI Center, forty New York City policemen and a dozen patrol cars greeted us, all assembled in front of the NYU offices. I knew my bilateral activation was a big deal—to me at least—but I didn't think it merited a full NYC police escort! But hey, why not! Maybe they had been tipped off!

Actually, I knew the real reason they were there. The United Nations is just a few blocks north and when there are bigwigs in the area, security is tight! These policemen were grouped in front of the

NYU building, most likely waiting for their assignments—but I like my version better.

Up we went to the seventh floor, sat down, and waited. These offices are so familiar to me now. There's usually someone I know having a mapping session, and today was no exception. I chatted briefly with a woman I recognized and ended up giving her information on how to get discounted tickets to the captioned performance of the Radio City Music Hall Christmas show—my good deed for the day.

Also sitting in the waiting room was a young woman I didn't recognize. She was there for some auditory therapy, and her therapist came out and told her that they were waiting for the interpreter to show up. *Hmmm*, I thought. I know who her interpreter is likely to be—my guardian angel of people with hearing loss at NYU, Jody! And sure enough, a few minutes later, in walked Jody—just the person who the very sight of brings calm and tranquility to my brain. Impeccable timing! I told her I was there for my bilateral activation and she came over to talk. She had just returned from a national hospital accreditation conference and was excited to tell me how she had been advocating for the needs of late-deafened and hard of hearing patients—just what we had discussed in the pre-op room before my CI surgery! Meanwhile, I was thinking to myself, "Oh my goodness . . . this bilateral surgery experience is starting to sprout wings!" But frankly, the timing—having my guardian angel appear at my first bilateral mapping. This was by chance?

By then, my audiologist had come into the waiting room, and we were ready for THE ACTIVATION! Betsy has been my audiologist from the beginning, so working with her is very familiar to me. As we began this session, I felt as if everything were moving in slow motion, taking forever to get to the crux of the matter: What was this processor going to sound like?

We started with the new ear alone, going through four sets of beeps—and I heard them! It was a little strange to hear with this ear. My brain was wondering what was going on. I had to decide what my comfort levels were for those beeps and I stayed very conservative in my responses. Betsy proceeded to make a program for me to try. Then came the moment of truth—that moment that I had been anticipating for months: turning on the processor. In the few seconds it took Betsy to switch on the processor, I said a very brief silent prayer. This is not something I routinely do, but that shows my state of mind. I needed some assistance on this!

And then we were on! Betsy sounded very high-pitched. My heart sank a little bit, but then I remembered my activation eleven years ago, and that things were weird in the beginning then, too. She kept talking, and then I realized that I could understand her. The more she talked, the more relaxed I got. I had understood speech at my activation eleven years ago, so I was hoping to do at least as well this time. We asked Ira to say a few words, and he sounded high-pitched as well. Not a surprise. It seems that because I hadn't heard high frequencies in decades, it was expected that everything would sound high-pitched in the beginning.

Betsy read four sentences out loud, then covered her mouth and repeated them one at a time. She asked me to repeat the sentence I heard. I got all of them correct! We proceeded to have a conversation, with no visual cues and only my new processor on. I could do that without a problem. Then she told me to put on the other ear's processor, so I would hear simultaneously with both ears. I did that, and the new processor sounded like a high-pitched echo, but it wasn't bothersome. She made me two other programs to try, packed up all my goodies to take home, and we were done for the day! I was exhausted.

I'm no novice at CIs and I knew right then and there that all I was going to do for the rest of the day was nothing! I wasn't going to try listening to music or test out new programs. I had no energy—mentally or physically—to do anything else. I even warned Ira not to test me, not to ask me how things sounded, but to just keep going through the rest of the day normally. I needed that—I knew my limits.

What did we do to continue the rest of the day normally? We put on the car's CD player. And what was in that CD player? The biography of Albert Einstein, the one that I had found too diffi-cult to listen to on the way to my activation appointment. And—I'm not making this up—it was not too difficult to listen to on the way home. I was absorbed in the dialogue—understanding it even with the road noise.

I had to laugh, though. Conventional wisdom for auditory therapy for new CI users is to start with books with simple dialogue—even children's books. And here I was sitting in the car with my brand-new CI and first hour of bilateral hearing, and what do I end up listening to? A discussion of Albert Einstein's special theory of relativity. Someone has a really good sense of humor, let me tell you!

Please don't ask me to explain what I was listening to! But I was getting the words, and there were some humdingers! There was no doubt that it was easier to understand with both processors on together. I briefly tried each processor separately, and it just wasn't as good as the two together.

I keep getting the impression that my new ear is like the baby sister getting dragged around by the big sister. It wants to be just like the other ear when it grows up!

My last task for the day was to mark the processors so I know which one is left and which one is right. And that is enough for one day.

OCTOBER 4, 2008 Two Ears/Two Days

The reality of having two ears is starting to sink in—not only because of the altered dynamics of hearing, but because I now have two sets of CI processors to contend with! That's not really something I thought too much about in the months anticipating bilateral hearing. I'm an old pro at putting the processor on my left side. My thick, curly hair is nicely tamped down at the magnet site, and I have no problem making my connections. Putting this new one on, though—that's a different story! It's like trying to write with my left hand. I don't have the coordination yet, and all those glorious curls make it incredibly difficult to even find the magnet site! The magnet on this processor is flush with my scalp, so there's hardly any telltale bump there. And my right hand has no clue what my left hand has been doing all these years! So this morning, it took me a little longer than one might expect just to get connected, but I suspect I'll get better at this! One thing I did learn—it's impossible to put the processor on the wrong ear. They're programmed not to work if that happens. Good thinking, guys!

I'm trying to be very casual about all this bilateral hearing. I really want to just get on with my life and not view this as another Mount Everest to be scaled, vying for records while doing so. Considering the events of the past several months, I have been through a lot—both mentally and physically—to the extent that I've started referring to this whole process as my CI decathlon! Going into this mapping, and the entire adaptation period, I've arrived at a mental attitude about the entire process. I'll do what I'm instructed to do, but I will not get into a frenzy of pushing myself to hear more/better/faster/sooner. With eleven years' experience of bionic hearing, I'm too much of a seasoned CI user to do that to myself. I have no deadlines to meet. In reality, the biggest goal was already met when that second set of electrodes was threaded into my cochlea. Now, if I hear more/better/ faster/sooner, that would be nice, but it's all icing on the cake. And frankly, I'm not so sure that heroic efforts beyond a calm, reasonable approach speed up the process, anyway.

I've now experienced almost two full days with bilateral hearing and I've passed the NYU CI Center's rite of passage of having two mappings in two days. My second mapping lacked the apprehension and fanfare that marked the initial activation. There was no New York City police escort greeting me at the entrance to the NYU building for this mapping session. Jody wasn't in the waiting room, either—guardian angels not required for this session. Getting set up was a lot easier, too—just hand over the processor, clip things on, and begin the mapping process. Betsy asked how I was doing, and I told her that I wore both processors and had no problems doing so. We then marched through the comfort level routine and I ended up increasing the volume on three of the four settings. When it was time to try this new program and see how it sounded, Betsy's voice sounded fuller. She was still high-pitched and robotic, but I could begin to detect a bit of what Betsy should really sound like. We had a conversation without visual cues, and she tested me on random sentences, also without visual cues, and I could understand it all. She then created two more programs, variations of the first. I now had three programs to try out and we were done.

I was instructed to wear both processors all the time. The only time I was supposed to wear the new processor alone was when I was doing auditory therapy—either with someone in professional therapy sessions or on my own at home. The rationale is to get the most practice using both ears together—the essential reason for going bilateral. I agreed with this approach because it dovetailed with my own agenda, which was to get on with my life. (Some CI centers recommend wearing the new CI processor alone for a month.) Adding that second ear didn't really change anything dramatically in my daily functioning since I could still hear at least as well with two ears as with one—that seems to be apparent. So I am not being put through the stress of trying to function with a brand-new ear alone, something I truthfully couldn't put myself through right now.

I got my car from the parking garage—bargain rates today because I got the early bird special—and off I went into my "mobile hearing testing lab." This felt very familiar. For all the times I've had mappings over the past eleven years, I was always eager to test out my new settings on the car's radio and CD player. Now I was in my comfort zone, not averse to trying out my new hearing with a variety of listening experiences.

I heard the news on the radio fine. I could hear it with both ears, sensing that slight echo effect coming from my new ear. Now I was curious about what my new ear would hear alone. I kept the news station on, and it sounded very thin, robotic, and high-pitched, as I expected. My brain was not keeping up with the words, but I felt if they just slowed down a bit, I could get it. I put my other ear back on, and it was as if the speech *had* slowed down—I understood it all, and there was a very rich timbre to the voices. I know that the speech on the radio hadn't slowed down just because I put my other ear on, but that is how my brain perceived it.

Music was next on my agenda. I figured I'd try my favorite jazz CD first. The last time I'd listened to it, the string bass was gone because the CI surgery had destroyed my low frequency residual hearing, but my brain had somehow rounded out the sound on its own, in whatever way brains can do that. I went right to "I Left My Heart in San Francisco," with the bluesy trumpet solo—and it was lovely! It was full, and I heard the tinkling of the piano keys in my new ear! I heard the sound of the trumpet in my new ear! I started to giggle. Now came the "new ear alone" test. I listened to that song again, and it was really strange. I could barely make out the sound of a piano, or a trumpet. I doubt I would have identified those instruments from what I was hearing. So I put my other ear back on—and there it all was again! Piano and trumpets in my new ear. *Hmmm . . .* Two ears together are *not* the sum of each ear individually—there's something else going on here!

I can only make a conjecture at this point in time—I've only been at this for less than forty-eight hours. But somehow, my brain is taking what it's hearing from the old ear, with its musical experience, and then taking what it's hearing from the new ear, and figuring out what it should be hearing. With the new ear on its own, my brain isn't really sure what it is hearing—but with the assistance of the other side, it can literally make music.

I called Ira on my cell phone to let him know I was on my way home. I could hear on the phone just as well as I had before—no change that I could discern. When I got home, Ira seemed incredibly happy. He just kept smiling at me, totally relieved that both CI surgeries were over and that my new hearing was going as well as anyone could expect. He was also wondering why I hadn't cried through any of this. He was right—I'm usually terrible at upheavals and new things. I get overwhelmed and just weep to let it all out. It may be because the support network that has surrounded me throughout this process has been so strong. It seemed that whenever I faltered, someone was there to keep me from toppling over. The truth is that I had cried briefly these past few days, but more with tears of gratitude and awe at getting through this incredible odyssey.

Keeping with my agenda to get on with my life, Ira and I went to the movies—captioned. No revelations there. I didn't feel I did any better or worse with both ears listening, and I chose a captioned movie so I wouldn't test myself. Afterward, we went out to eat at one of the most cacophonous restaurants imaginable: high ceilings, marble floors, wall-to-wall tables teeming with people, plus piped-in music. I had no trouble hearing Ira through this. As a matter of fact, I was doing so well that the surrounding horrendous noise levels weren't registering to me as horrendous noise levels at all.

It was so loud, though, that I realized I was raising my voice to be heard. I immediately pulled off my new ear and listened with my old one—cacophonous noise! I put back my new ear. Much better! I know they told me that being bilateral would allow me to do better in noise, but I figured I would have to learn to use my new ear first, and also learn to use my two ears together. I'm sure I'm a quick study with all this, but not that quick! Evidently, when the brain has another ear functioning—even a brand-new ear—it does better in noise.

OCTOBER 7, 2008 Stereo

As a seasoned CI user, having adapted to new processors twice, I feel confident and comfortable charting my own course. I know myself well, too. Although the objectives are obvious—adapt to the new ear and merge both ears together—there is a third objective: make sure not to burn myself out or end up hating all this. I have already heard from a well-intentioned professional who assumed that I was "hard at work practicing my listening skills." No! No! No! That is *not* what I'm doing now! I'm having fun exploring having two ears!

I'm using two processors all the time now, but for auditory therapy, I'm letting my new ear play with sound on its own briefly each day. Even though this ear started out understanding speech without visual cues, everything sounded like a high-pitched robot, and environmental sounds began as mere swishes. Even now, when I put the processor on, all I hear for the first few moments is an electronic hoot. The first order of business, then, is to tame the environment, so I've devoted breakfast time to listening with my new ear alone. I feel this is the right approach because it is similar to the philosophy of having toddlers learn by playing, not by pushing them to read!

I'm astounded at how quickly this ear is learning! Two days ago, my footsteps were just electronic whistles. Now they're footsteps. And just as a toddler explores his world of sound by playing with a pot and a spoon, I've been listening to the clatter of dishes, glasses, and silverware as I unload the dishwasher each morning. I've been putting on the television, too. Two days ago I could follow and understand some of an interview program, but none of the news. Today I could follow some of the news that eluded me the day before. I also test Ira's voice each morning, and it has started to come down in pitch. And one of the traditional CI rites of passage—the toilet flushing—is also sounding less and less like Niagara Falls!

There is still a long way to go, but I'm happy, and that is a significant part of my plan. I don't think a non-CI user can appreciate the upheaval I've endured these past seven months—the silence, the surgeries, the adaptations, the fears, the expectations. I've been tenacious in getting to this point and now that I've gotten a brief glimpse at what I've been given to work with, I'm ready to have fun! I also feel like an elder statesman, and trust my own judgment that this is the right way to proceed for now.

The morning time devoted to just one ear is the only special attention I've been giving to this bilateral process. For everything else, two ears are now the norm. Each day, it seems, I discover a little more.

I attended a bridal shower over the weekend—my first time socializing in a group. The first thing I realized was that I no longer have to put everyone on my left side! Actually, Ira discovered this on day one. He started to walk on my left side, but then realized that he didn't have to anymore. Poor guy, for the past thirty-five years, as I switched hearing aids and then the CI processor, first to the left, then to the right, and then back to the left again, he had to remember which was my "better side." No more. I'm "normal" again!

At the bridal shower, I was mindful of being kind to myself, getting a feel for the environment before plunging into conversations. I opted to sit and talk with my daughter and her friend, rather than seat myself at a round table for eight, which I felt would be too stressful for my first time out with two ears. I was generally doing fine—not as carefree as the hearing people there, but not struggling, either. Emily informed me that there was background music, which I couldn't really discern, and that the noise level wasn't bad, just moderate. I was curious how things would sound without my new ear, so I pulled off the magnet. I was astonished at the difference! Everything was blending together—even Emily's voice, and she was sitting right in front of me! It may be utterly cliché to say this, but it really was like the difference between seeing in two dimensions rather than three! With both processors on, Emily's voice sounded close, and the other noise was relegated to the background. No surprise—that's what I had thought hearing in noise would be like. But experiencing it in person was eye-opening!

I had driven to this bridal shower on my own, so I was looking forward to some adventures in my "mobile hearing testing lab" on the way home. I felt it was my duty to listen to some speech, but I really was itching to listen to my jazz CD again. That's when things got interesting.

I noticed that I could hear the piano and trumpet in my new ear. But I realized that I *wasn't* hearing the piano and trumpet in my *old* ear. *Hmmm* . . . How could that be? I knew that my old ear could hear pianos and trumpets very well. Then it dawned on me—I must be hearing *in stereo.*

And the jazz sounded good! I was hearing the melody with my new ear on the right, and the accompaniment with my old ear on the left. What's perplexing, though, is that my new ear doesn't have the capability to hear those instruments that well! It can hear pianos and trumpets, but they sound a little warpy and meek, yet I was perceiving them through this new ear just the way my old ear would have. What seems to be happening is that I now have enough hearing in my new ear to trigger some "two ear" responses in my brain. Actually, I'm not at all sure just what is happening!

I surmise that hearing people think they're only hearing from the ear on the side a sound is coming from. But my experience with this stereo jazz CD seems to be different—my brain is commandeering my right ear and making it seem to me that all the sounds both ears are picking up that are emanating from the right speaker are being heard by my right ear. Whatever—I come out the winner, because my poor little new ear that just woke up four days ago already thinks it can hear sophisticated jazz harmony! All the more reason to keep listening with two ears.

A similar experience occurred when I watched TV that evening. I'm not much of a TV watcher, but I decided to join Ira, watching *CSI: Miami*. As the show progressed, I noticed that I was hearing some eerie background music all around me. We have a Bose surround sound system in our TV room. It never meant much to me, because with one ear, it all sounded as if it were coming from the front. I asked Ira, is there eerie music coming from all different directions in this room? And he said yes! Who knew? I guess it didn't make any sense to bring it up if I couldn't hear the difference, anyway. Now—oh my goodness—I was surrounded by a swirl of ethereal music. I've never experienced anything like it. It was magical! Surround sound didn't even exist the last time I had two functioning ears! I immediately did a reality check, pulling off the magnet on my new ear, and the swirling music stopped—like a mirage, it was gone!

I put my new ear back on, and the music was back, coming from the speakers around me. It seems that my brain had gone into "two ear mode" again, and my new ear was being used to perceive sounds that it never would have been able to on its own. I still can't quite believe it!

There's no doubt in my mind now that human beings were made to have two ears. Our brains are wired for it.

OCTOBER 10, 2008 Days of Awe

I've made it through my first week with two processors, and that is something to celebrate! The first week with a new CI is usually the hardest—the expectations, the nervousness, the uncertainty, those first sounds, and living with new sounds every waking moment. This is my third time breaking in a new processor, so I at least had the advantage of having a basic idea what to expect. But this listening situation—adapting to a new ear and merging it with an existing ear—

presents a unique challenge. I'm very heartened that my plans to tackle this—adapting while considering my emotional well-being—have gotten me off to a good start!

What has surprised me the most so far is that my own voice, with only the new processor on, sounds almost normal now—so soon! There's a robotic quality to it, but I'm delighted to hear all the consonants crisply articulated. The merge with my other ear is going nicely, too. I'm not having difficulty wearing both processors together, though I still hear a little high-pitched echo coming from the new processor. One quirk is that if I take off my old ear to momentarily check how my new ear is doing, the new ear sounds as primitive as day one again. So whatever it has learned so far when combined with the old ear hasn't "stuck" yet when it's on its own.

This past week overlaid exactly the time period between Rosh Hashanah and Yom Kippur, traditionally called the "Days of Awe." It's a time for introspection, looking back on the past year, and gathering thoughts and hopes for the approaching new year. That's a pretty apt description for this past week with my new processor as well!

I even had a chance to perform "good deeds," or charity this week—traditional, along with prayer and repentance, during these Days of Awe. It always seems to be about hearing, though. I was asked for advice on how to help a ninety-year-old woman struggling with hearing loss, what a twelve-year-old who had just lost most of his hearing should do, and I gave my older CI body-worn processor, the one I could no longer use, to another CI user who needed it.

My family attended services on the evening of Yom Kippur, called Kol Nidre. It's during that service that the cantor chants the melodious Kol Nidre prayer, asking forgiveness for past sins and transgressions. It had become a tradition in my temple to have a cellist also play this mournful tune. My mother had been a cellist and had played this melody as I was growing up, so I have deep emotional associations with it. As we entered the sanctuary, I was disappointed to discover that there would be no cellist this year, but a string bass player instead. That was an interesting turn of events! My father, who had been a high school instrumental music teacher and could play all the instruments in the orchestra, had played string bass professionally. I seemed to be trading one emotional attachment for another! Yet the string bass was the one instrument that I thought I couldn't hear anymore on my jazz CD because the CI surgery had effectively destroyed my low frequency hearing. How was I supposed to hear this string bass? The answer seemed to be staring straight at me: Have faith!

I knew it would help to sit up close, so I could see the instrument being played and hear it directly, not through loudspeakers. As the bassist began to play, I watched and I listened. My old ear was picking up low frequency sounds—some VERY low frequency sounds. I don't know why I could hear it in front of me but not on my CD—that still remains a mystery. My new ear couldn't hear those low frequencies, but was hearing the melody higher pitched. So my old ear heard what sounded like a string bass, and my new ear heard what sounded like a cello! I could follow the melody since I knew what they were playing, but the sounds didn't mingle. It was as if two instruments were playing, and my emotions were being tugged by both.

As the services continued, I had my assistive listening device standing by in case I needed it. I didn't. I was doing better at this service with two ears than I had at last week's Rosh Hashanah service with one—and again, it sounded better without the headset than with it. Sitting up front was helpful, as I was able to hear the rabbi, cantor and choir directly, not through the loudspeakers. I noticed that when the choir sang, I seemed to be able to tell who was singing the solo parts. I was never able to do that before. In years past, I would scan the choir members' faces to see whose mouth was moving! Presumably, some sort of directionality was now coming into play. I also sensed that the rabbi, cantor, and choir members were noticing that I wasn't using the headset very much. I caught their eyes once or twice and felt them silently cheering me on!

The part of the service I was looking forward to the most came last: the blowing of the shofar. This marks the official end of the old year and the start of the new. Five shofars were blown simultaneously—one unified sound that was loud, piercing, and wonderful!

Reflecting back on the events leading up to this moment, the timing was once again impeccable, as if this had been the objective all along—to hear the blowing of the shofar on Yom Kippur with two ears. It signaled the end of a year that saw my hearing dramatically transformed and heralded the start of a new year and a new journey.

OCTOBER 17, 2008   Finding Happiness

Happy. I guess that's how you'd describe my mood after two weeks using two ears. I'll give some specifics, but those are almost beside the point. I just like hearing with two ears, as imperfect, new, and ever-changing as it is! I couldn't have imagined this when I first contemplated going bilateral.

From the start, it was apparent that I could function at least as well with two ears as I had with one, so I had the luxury of playing with the sounds. No pressure. No diagnostic testing. No intense practice sessions. Just letting my natural curiosity explore, allowing me time to recover fully from the trauma of surgery and the newness of another processor.

My objective has been to let my new ear wake up gently on its own, and that strategy seems to be agreeing with me. What began as a high-pitched robotic sound has started to evolve, with lower frequencies emerging. When I put the processor on in the morning, I no longer hear a high-pitched electronic hoot. My nerve has gotten used to being stimulated. And that Einstein biography CD—the one with the special theory of relativity I listened to on my very first day using two ears—has started to evolve as well. I just listened again, first with two ears and then with just my new one. The narrator's voice sounds deep to my new ear, still robotic but clearer. Those lows are starting to come in now!

I'm noticing subtle differences using two ears that would never be apparent to someone who hasn't experienced one-sided hearing. I was on a guided tour of an historic house, the homestead of the Arts and Crafts movement's adherent, Gustav Stickley. The tour guide had a deep voice, which I was finding very easy to understand.

When I had one processor, I would usually position myself so that my better side was closer to the guide. That wasn't necessary now, and there was a calmness that felt new to me. I wasn't working to hear or figuring out the best logistics. I tried listening with one ear, and I immediately sensed a tension—my brain going on higher alert to field the sounds. Everything sounded flatter and less vibrant that way. With two ears, the sounds just flowed in. I found myself responding quickly to questions, or injecting my own comments. I know I've described this when using just one new processor—and I certainly thought I was doing quite well with that processor, but this is different. The difference is subtle, but definite. It's more natural and, the best way to describe it—normal.

I'm also getting more accustomed to the idea that I don't have a "better side" anymore. I don't have to sit on the right side of a car or at the right end of a table or maneuver to the right side of the people I'm with. They say that when an action is repeated twelve times, it becomes a habit. Is twelve times all it takes to undo thirty-five years of one-sided indoctrination? Hard to believe, but that's really what has been happening. If anything, I'm making sure that my new ear is given a little extra chance to get practice—putting it closer to the speaker if I feel like it. It's still weak when sound is coming from only that side, but otherwise the two ears are working together.

This twelve-time habit-breaking theory seems to apply to my listening preferences, too. After twelve days of putting on two processors, I've started to get used to hearing with two ears. I still do my early morning breakfast routine using only my new ear, to give it a chance to build itself up, but other than that, I'm becoming accustomed to hearing with two ears. Without my new ear listening in, my brain is sensing that something is missing now.

I'm also feeling more in command of my environment, or more *connected*. What I'm hearing is far from perfect, and there are times when I need repeats, and the noise level can still be too much, or there are too many people speaking at once. But I seem to stay calmer, as if the solutions are as simple as making a few adjustments. There's a lack of "frantic," or "worry," or "thinking to hear." Again, it's subtle.

A good example is my birthday dinner two days ago—a table for fourteen in a quiet restaurant environment. That, in itself, should have produced immediate tension. I can't expect to hear everyone at a table for fourteen, but I wasn't tense. I chose a seat in the middle, and why I didn't worry about hearing everyone at the table, I still can't quite figure out. I was happy to hear the person on my right, and on my left, and even beyond. When the conversation turned to others across the table, I got some of it, and sometimes I'd ask for help, but my general demeanor was that this situation was not going to overwhelm me, nor would I need to retreat. I was more in command and I liked the way that felt.

I've been revisiting my stereo listening experiences. I'm not sure now that I've been hearing music in true stereo. But does it matter? I know that I'm hearing music in both ears, and each ear hears something a little different when listening together. The crux of the matter is that the two ears together always sound better! Whether that's technically "stereo"—well, for a deaf person, we shouldn't have to split hairs on this—at least not after only two weeks!

I didn't think my happy feelings were tied to specifics, but doing a quick recap, there do seem to be some compelling reasons: I'm no longer one-sided, music sounds better, I feel more in command, and my hearing, in general, has improved. Those are all good reasons for me to feel happy. But the real reason is probably something subtler: I sense that my brain has finally found the ear it has been searching for all these years.

OCTOBER 23, 2008   Revelations

This bilateral journey is starting to get more interesting! I've learned that using the phone while having two ears presents some new and novel challenges! When I'm talking on the phone using my old ear, my own voice now sounds different. That shouldn't really be a surprise: I'm now hearing my voice with two ears, but it still seems a little strange to me. I'm also hearing more environmental sounds when on the phone, and that can be intrusive! The solution was not hard to figure out: I just pull off the magnet on my other ear and the noise stops. The benefits of being bionic!

It also occurred to me that my old ear is not getting much practice listening alone, which is still the skill it needs to use the phone. I'm now making sure to use the phone each day, even if it's just calling 800 numbers. I want that ear to continue functioning optimally on its own.

I've been hesitant to try the phone with my new ear. The issue was forced on me this week, though. As I was talking to my daughter, the battery in my old ear died. I had the choice of either replacing the battery (the wimp option) or switching ears (the very essence of being bilateral). I stared at the phone receiver for what seemed like forever, and then switched ears. Something about holding the phone in my right hand felt strangely familiar. It's something I grew up doing. And I didn't do too badly! Emily, with her native New Jersey mile-a-minute speech, slowed down for me, and we were able to converse. I'm not ready to declare myself a switch phone-user yet, but now I think I'll give that ear some phone practice, too.

I've been on the lookout for some evidence of directional hearing. I'd really love to turn my head to a loud sound, or something that would dramatically prove that my brain can tell which side sounds are coming from. That just hasn't happened yet. No epiphanies.

I had the opportunity to show off my cochlear implant processor this week. I've found that many people have heard of CIs, but most have never actually seen one. As I was giving one of my CI mini-lessons, I removed my right processor, and nothing changed! I could still hear myself talking! When I had only one processor, I'd ask people if my voice changed as I explained the processor, since I would then be totally without sound. Not anymore! I'm going to have to think this over. That was always such a poignant demonstration of the correlation between hearing oneself and voice quality. With a second ear, my demo just got a little less exciting, dramatic, and informative. Not to worry—it's a problem I don't mind having.

OCTOBER 26, 2008 Better in Noise

It's only been three weeks using two ears, and I know that I'm still at the very beginning of the adaptation process. That's why I am so bewildered to find so much benefit from bilateral hearing so soon. I am totally convinced, once again, that we were made to have two ears. It matters.

Just this weekend I attended two parties: a surprise birthday party and an early Halloween party, both very noisy. Just as I was led to expect, I did do better in noise using both ears. But those words, *better in noise*, sitting here on the page, don't begin to do justice to the experience.

I had preconceived ideas about what doing "better in noise" would mean. I expected socializing to be easier, that I wouldn't have to maneuver people to my good side or away from the noisiest areas to talk. That's what I thought, and I was correct, but the reality is much more complex.

Being able to do better in noise changes the experience itself. During the birthday party, I endured three hours of listening in noise—a large room with fifty people talking, six televisions tuned to different stations, and piped-in background music. As noisy as this was, it was as if I had been sprinkled with pixie dust that made me visible, outgoing, and conversant! As the evening wore on, I was waiting to get stressed out or tire of navigating this situation, but it never happened. And, yes, even my husband was wondering when I was going to "tune out," and was also surprised that I didn't. I really do hesitate to say I felt as if I had normal hearing—it doesn't rise to that. But I was astonished to hear comments from around our table and the give-and-take as the presents were being opened. I was an active participant, commenting and joking with everyone else. I didn't hear some people from a few feet behind me, but I was getting so much, it was changing my behavior. I was like someone else—or some new, improved version of myself.

The Halloween party had over a hundred people—rambunctious, shrieking kids and their parents—all in a small suburban household (not mine!). The same thing happened at this party as the other one—all that noise, but it was basically not intruding on the experience. It was as if the noise was somehow controlled, tamed, put into place. Just like my birthday dinner last week, I felt more in command—and with that feeling, my behavior and body language changed.

It wasn't perfect, of course—the close proximity to a lot of children did present listening challenges, but the other adults also commented on the noise level. So doing better in noise may sound like a simple, noble objective, but as is often the case with hearing loss, the practical impact goes far deeper than one might expect. It certainly caught me off guard that it could change my experience so greatly—making me feel much less hearing impaired. I liked that.

I've been very pleased with my decision not to go headlong into formal auditory therapy sessions. The three weeks I've spent playing with my new hearing have been so right for me! I let my natural curiosity try out all sorts of sounds without the pressure or stress of having to listen to word lists or be accountable to anyone. I really needed this time to get acquainted with my new ear. It reminds me of how I raised my children, backing off on formal music lessons when I saw that it was threatening their love of music. Later on, both my children asked for lessons because they wanted to go further with their musical interests. And that is what seems to have happened with my new ear, too. I've had my chance to explore, and now I feel the need for some professional guidance. Fortunately, NYU has auditory therapy available in the same location as my mapping sessions, so I simply arranged for appointments on the same day as my next two mappings. I'm completely comfortable with this setup now, but three weeks ago, it was too much for me to even contemplate.

I have also continued to explore on my own, listening to the MP3 files and videos that are cropping up on the *New York Times* website. This gives me additional impromptu listening practice right at my desk—and a worthwhile way to procrastinate! But it does make this kind of practice a natural extension of my daily routine, and I like that approach.

With all this attention focused on my hearing, it is no surprise that these experiences made their way into my dreams. I've had this happen before. When I first started to lose my hearing, I became hard of hearing in my dreams as well. That was so upsetting to me—I couldn't even catch a break in my sleep! My latest dream, last night, was the exact opposite! In it, I was moving through a roomful of people, casually answering questions without much effort. Doing better in noise—even in my dreams.

OCTOBER 31, 2008 Playing for Real

I attended another arts access task force meeting, the state Council on the Arts committee I have been involved with for almost fifteen years. I hadn't requested assistive listening devices or real-time captioning because I had done very well with my single new processor at the last meeting. This time, there were seven of us around a table. The room had bare floors and windows, and a bit of an echo. I had taken a seat "anywhere"—not right or left—because I could!

As discussions started, I knew right away that this was different—and my brain knew it, too. I was just hearing—and not like the last meeting with one processor. I was really hearing—without effort, and differently. My brain was telling me "this is the way you used to hear." This time, I won't hesitate to say that this sounded like normal hearing. It did. I wasn't only hearing and understanding the words. I sensed where the voices were in relation to the rest of the room. And not only that, I was turning to the person speaking—right, left, and ahead. I couldn't quite believe this was happening, so I let the meeting continue, listening and talking. Then I tried listening with just my new ear, curious about the sound quality. I was surprised that the voices with just the new ear had pretty much the same pitch range as the two ears together—just more nasal and robotic.

Of course, I announced that I was hearing really well with my two ears, but everyone already knew that. I was responding so quickly, it was apparent to me that this was not just *better*, but *real* hearing. I can't say that I remember what real hearing was like, but I know my brain remembers. It has demonstrated its long-term auditory memory before.

Now I'm wondering what was special about this situation, because this is the first time I've had this feeling of normal hearing. It must have helped that it was a small meeting. I wasn't overwhelmed and there wasn't any extraneous noise. I've also been reading about bilateral hearing, and evidently you need a certain range of frequencies for certain properties of bilateral hearing to kick in. This may correlate with what I've just reported, that my new ear has filled in the low frequencies and is starting to sound more natural.

Believe it or not, I did not turn on the radio during the entire trip home. For some reason, I wanted to stay in the zone and think this over.

NOVEMBER 25, 2008 Practice and Progress

I feel as though I've just completed the eight-week course, *Introduction to Bilateral Cochlear Implants 101*! When I first went bilateral, I knew to expect four probable outcomes: general improvement in hearing, better functioning in noise, eventual improvement in directionality, and a general sense of happiness hearing with two ears. While all this is accurate, it seems a little simplistic now that I've had a chance to experience bilateral CI hearing firsthand—in depth and personal! It is so much more complex than I ever expected that I now sense that there are stages, and I've just passed the first one. This is my description of the "introductory course":

> **INTRODUCTION TO BILATERAL COCHLEAR IMPLANTS 101:**
> This eight-week course will enable you to explore a variety of listening experiences using your new cochlear implant processor alone and in conjunction with your existing one. Emphasis will be on keeping the entire process relaxed and enjoyable. Listening practice will focus on the sounds of everyday activities, with materials determined by the interests of the student. The course will conclude with an auditory therapy session, when the new ear will be evaluated, and practice materials for the next course will be discussed.

The final exam will consist of the following essay question: What is an unexpected characteristic of bilateral CI hearing that no person with normal hearing will ever experience? Provide two examples.

Here's my answer to the final exam question, just in time for Thanksgiving break!

An unexpected characteristic of bilateral CI hearing is that even if the new ear doesn't sound very good on its own yet and is still in the process of improving its speech discrimination, it can still supply the brain with enough volume and frequency range to allow it to create an alternate reality—the bilateral functioning of two ears, while seeming to sound at least as good as the better ear. A person with normal hearing in both ears has no way to know that the brain can do this "sleight of sound."

This is so amazing to experience! I had this happen just last week when my husband and I took my son out to dinner for his birthday. His wife couldn't come, so it was just the three of us at a table for four at a lovely French restaurant. I immediately realized that the walls and floors were hard surfaces, so the acoustics were not the best. Then I noticed that a group of women was being seated to the right of our table—a sure source of unwelcome noise. But we were there for the five-course tasting menu, something we were really looking forward to. There was no turning back now!

With my son on my right, he was near my new ear, so I just assumed that I would hear him with the rather robotic sound quality that ear still has. But that's not what happened. My son sounded normal. And not just normal—I could hear his voice separately from the background noise coming from the other table. I could also hear my husband on my left, also normal-sounding. I was simply hearing—not with the left ear or the right ear, or trying to block out noise. I had all the benefits of bilateral hearing, with normal speech sounds, even though the new ear doesn't hear like that alone.

I had a similar experience this past weekend while visiting with friends. We were dabbling with their computer. I was sitting at the desk and my friend was sitting on a chair, positioned behind my right shoulder. She was as far from my old ear as could be, yet when we spoke with each other, I could understand her quite well without looking, and she sounded normal. With my new ear alone, her high female voice would probably have sounded like a chipmunk robot. But with both ears, her voice was as normal as it had always sounded to me. Again, my bilateral hearing enabled me to hear *better*, and with normal speech sounds, even though the new ear doesn't sound that good alone yet.

It is really counterintuitive—how the brain can simultaneously benefit from the input of the new ear while making it seem as good as the old ear. Anyone with normal hearing would have no way to know this is even possible.

That answers the final exam question, but it makes one wonder whether it's really worth working so hard to improve the function of the new ear if the brain does so well with its less-than-perfect incarnation? The answer, of course, is that I won't really know until I find out for myself. That's the next course—*Bilateral Hearing at the Intermediate Level*! The task at hand is to choose the appropriate practice materials.

At my first auditory therapy session, we determined that the materials I had already been using—phone practice, online videos, captioned television, car radio—were still very effective at giving me the practice I needed, and I was given website addresses that had additional practice resources to explore. Eleven years ago, my auditory therapy consisted of listening to books on tape. I had one body processor, which had a jack, and I used a "patch cord" to connect to a Walkman tape player. I also listened to the tapes in my car. I thought this was so cutting-edge, but it is practically monastic living compared to the myriad choices I'm facing now! How to choose? Essentially, going back to my original philosophy of listening practice—find a listening routine that I'm comfortable with that is quick and easy to access.

I continue to enjoy watching the videos that crop up on the news websites—some are captioned, some are not. Internet videos are good because they can be repeated easily and listened to with each ear separately or both together. And current events videos are actually a useful learning tool, beneficial beyond hearing practice. They're *real*. I like that.

I also like the practice websites that have word lists and diagnostic testing. I've learned that my new ear's speech discrimination is actually quite good! I never wanted to be tested before. It usually stresses me out to be graded like that. But now, after eight weeks, I've calmed down, and this word list regimen seems like a good way to track my "personal best" progress.

I've also found phone practice very beneficial because it brings the sound directly into the microphone of my processor. Sound that goes directly in like that, in my experience, has usually been the most potent in beating pathways to the brain. Phone practice also addresses the emotional baggage of using the phone. The simple act of picking up the receiver reinforces an I'm-able-to-do-this-now feeling.

The ultimate challenge, though, is Thanksgiving, a holiday that is centered around one of the most difficult listening environments: a large dinner table. I'm no novice when it comes to the coping strategies designed to navigate this minefield, but this year, maybe, just maybe, my bilateral powerhouse processors will carry me through.

NOVEMBER 29, 2008 The First Thanksgiving

I'm smiling. I had a wonderful Thanksgiving. I had such high hopes that my bilateral powerhouse processors would carry me through this holiday, and they did. We conquered Thanksgiving and I'm still savoring the experience!

Thanksgiving is probably the most difficult day on the calendar for someone with a hearing loss. It looks innocent enough—a welcoming family environment, smiling faces, laughter, conversation, comfort food. For someone with a hearing loss, though, the main activity is typically watching other people talk to one another and, at sporadic moments, wondering why everyone else is laughing heartily. There are gradations of this, of course, with varying degrees of hearing, assistive equipment, and coping strategies—but it's not the holiday everyone else is having. You're supposed to feel happy and grateful, yet that's virtually impossible if you have to struggle to communicate. The stress, the conflicting emotions—it's not hard to imagine that Thanksgiving feels like something to be conquered.

So how did bilateral processors make such a difference for me? When I first arrived at my niece's house, I headed straight to the kitchen and sat down at the counter. My niece was at the sink, my sister-in-law was on my right, and a football game was playing at low volume on the television behind me. We had a three-way conversation, even with the water running and the football noise. Other people came into the kitchen, and I not only watched them have a conversation, I heard what they were saying. I don't even remember what they were talking about. It wasn't very important. I do remember, though, how sad it can feel to watch conversations without knowing what is being said. Being able to hear even inconsequential conversations has an emotional impact. This time I felt involved and connected.

The real challenge, of course, came when we sat down to dinner. My niece was hosting twenty-two people at an L-shaped table. I didn't have to worry about who would get my better side, since both sides are good now. Sitting "anywhere" still feels new and liberating! I could hear conversations going on to my right, and also down at the other end of the table. It was a curious feeling—very new to me. I could place all the conversations. It wasn't a blur of background noise.

We had a bountiful meal—most likely more food than any Pilgrim ever saw—so conversation at that point was simply "pass this" and "pass that." But I was connected even to those mundane interactions—some from the left, some from the right, and even some behind me—and all that counts, too. Then, after all the chewing had subsided, the chatting began. I'm still smiling thinking about what happened next.

I struck up a conversation with my daughter-in-law, who was sitting diagonally across the table from me. While we were talking, Ira was having an animated conversation with his sister, who was directly across the table from me. Their conversation was actually flying over mine. People were conversing to my right and there was a conversation going on at the other end of the table, where all the children were. The fact that I could hold a conversation across a table under these conditions was mind-boggling. My bilateral powerhouse processors were working their magic!

Ira noticed right away that I was having a conversation across the table and knew this was a very significant moment. He hadn't seen me hold a conversation like that since I started losing my hearing. I'd had short "coping conversations," totally controlled by the myriad strategies in my bag of hearing tricks to make it appear as though I were functioning like everyone else. But that's not what was happening here. I wasn't using any coping strategies, other than to have the good fortune of having bilateral cochlear implant processors assisting me.

That's not quite accurate, either. It's not just about the two processors. Sure, there is no way that one processor alone could possibly be as effective as two, even with the best noise management algorithms. But what this is also about is what happens when that second processor comes on board. It evidently activates a specific area of the brain whose task is to coordinate the sounds coming into both ears. It doesn't simply add the sound input from the second side. The brain actually lays out a sound landscape, like a 3-D site plan. It's as if I had a map with a key identifying the locations of the sounds surrounding me. With one ear, that isn't possible, as all sounds seem to come from one location and blend together. That 3-D site plan is the key to conquering Thanksgiving!

Before my first CI, it was impossible to communicate at Thanksgiving on any effective level, so I usually didn't even bother. I couldn't. At my first Thanksgiving with a CI ten years ago, I was in such awe of being able to hear again, I didn't focus on its shortcomings. It was too much of a miracle to quibble over details. But in subsequent years, I did face the realities of one-sided hearing and noise management, and developed various coping strategies. Those strategies served me well, but they required forethought and effort just to remain connected.

This Thanksgiving, as I took off my two processors that night, I was swept up by emotion. I know that my bilateral hearing is still not normal hearing, but it was close enough that Thanksgiving this year was not about struggling or coping strategies—it was about feeling happy and grateful. It stirred fond memories from long ago, before hearing loss intruded on this family tradition. These thoughts bring tears to my eyes. This was truly a Thanksgiving homecoming.

DECEMBER 7, 2008 Intermediate Level

I finally made it to my exercise class—the first time since my surgery on September 10. I guess that means I'm officially recovered. I'm not sure what was taking me so long. I just hadn't felt ready until now. I was welcomed back with open arms! My classmates were all relieved to learn that "good things" had kept me away.

I was very curious to see what difference two ears would make in that big room with high ceilings, bare floors, and large stereo speakers. As soon as the exercise music began, I could tell the difference immediately. I was hearing it up close and loud, much louder than I had ever heard this music before. I asked Janet, the instructor, if the volume was higher than usual, and she said it wasn't. This was supposed to be background music, but for me, it was anything but!

During the class, not that much had changed in my speech comprehension. I could still understand Janet as she guided us through our "marching orders." About ten minutes into the class, it dawned on me that I no longer needed Janet on my left side. I had been taking that spot for so long—years, in fact—that the reasons for doing so had slipped my mind! How could it possibly slip my mind that I could now hear from either side? Old habits die hard!

I had hoped to hear the ongoing banter better—there's always a running conversation between Janet and the members of the class. I did hear the other people talking, but without looking at them—and even with looking at them—I still wasn't able to follow much of what they were saying. It was a big room, though, with bad acoustics and music playing, so I really shouldn't be too disappointed.

One surprise, besides the loudness of the background music, was the sound of people putting down their weights. I had never heard this as a specific sound before, only as general background noise, but now it was all over the room, weights dropping as we changed exercises! That was my bilateral "hearing better in noise" kicking in—in a totally useless way! I imagine that everyone in the class had tuned this sound out by now, but for me, it was brand-new! I guess my brain didn't realize that these thuds and clunks weren't important to me. I'm still such a novice at this!

By the end of the hour, I had yet another surprise. The background music that had been "up close and loud" when the session began was now quiet in the background, where it belonged. This is so strange. How could my brain figure out that this sound was supposed to be in the background after listening for only an hour? I'm starting to think that in *Bilateral Hearing at the Intermediate Level*, I've just advanced to the next chapter—managing background sounds. The fact that I had a similar experience just a few days later seems to reinforce my theory.

I was in Macy's doing some shopping when I heard piped-in music very clearly and much louder than I had ever heard it before. It was so clear that I even understood some of the "Christmas Eve" lyrics, pretty incredible for some inconsequential background music! It was incessant, though! Christmas music followed me everywhere in that store, including into the fitting room. This would really have been humorous if it wasn't so annoying. It was as if I now had *two* high quality CD players in my head, broadcasting nonstop, in stereo. When I went to pay for my purchases, I asked the cashier if the music was particularly loud. She replied that she had tuned it out so long ago, she didn't even notice it anymore! I wasn't about to stick around for an hour to find out if my brain was going to relegate this background music to its rightful place. My hunch, though, is that it probably would have!

I've continued to practice my listening skills—left, right, and together. We tend to focus on the together part, but the individual ears are important as well. People with normal hearing don't always use two ears together. They also hear with each ear individually—getting whispers or talking on the phone—and I want to do what hearing people do with two ears! I'm enjoying this practice regimen so much that I now find myself using the phone and word exercises as an excuse to procrastinate doing my other tasks! This is an interesting turn of events—practice materials I had considered too arduous and structured to tackle at the beginning of this bilateral journey have now become my playthings! That, in itself, proves that my instincts were right on target about what practice materials to choose.

And I continue to feel happy about having two ears, a fortuitous quirk of this bilateral experience. I don't recall having this same type of emotion when I only had one processor. Yes, of course, I have always been enormously happy to be able to hear again—actually thrilled, grateful, and in awe of this miracle every single day—but that's not the same as this contented little feeling of just being happy to hear with both ears. I've met people who had suddenly lost their hearing in one ear, and they are often disoriented and upset. Maybe what I'm experiencing with my second ear restored is the opposite of those intense emotions. Whatever the reason, I'm enjoying this bilateral world. Even the raindrops sound better here.

DECEMBER 11, 2008 Sound Decisions

This week's plans were made months ago—four appointments squeezed into three days, all related to my bilateral CI. Monday was a mapping and auditory therapy session. Wednesday was the three-month evaluation, scheduled a bit early at ten weeks. And Thursday was the post-op appointment with my surgeon. It was the CI evaluation that had motivated me to do so much listening practice, so I was particularly looking forward to that.

It turns out that life is not a dress rehearsal, and listening practice is actually geared to functioning in real-life situations, not soundproof booths. I got my reality check Wednesday morning on the trip into the city for my evaluation. I was coming off the George Washington Bridge and took the turn off the exit ramp a little too close, scraping my front right tire on the curb. I heard the metallic sound (with both ears) and gasped, hoping that I hadn't done any permanent damage to the tire. But then I heard a grinding sound coming from that side of the car and felt the vibration in my steering wheel. My stress level started to rise, because upper Manhattan was a bad place to have car problems. Conventional wisdom says that a woman driving alone does not stop or get out of her car there. I had no choice but to keep driving. I made sure I could still steer and that my brakes still worked.

I was hoping that my tire would make it to the parking garage near the NYU CI Center at 38th Street, seven miles away. As I drove, louder, raspy clunking sounds began to come from the right front side of my car. Fortunately, traffic had slowed down to a crawl. I called my husband and then NYU on my cell phone to let them know what was happening. Several people passing me in their cars were pointing to my tire, so I figured it was flat by now. When traffic started moving faster, I definitely heard metal scraping against the road. I was driving on the rim. I knew I had to get off the highway (there were no shoulders), so I finally exited at 96th Street in an area that was fairly busy. I parked by a fire hydrant and called AAA.

Now I was glad I had practiced using the phone separately with both ears. It ensured that my old ear had kept up its phone proficiency, and it also gave me more confidence to do this under stress—and I was under stress! The AAA dispatcher was a pro and he knew his territory. I'm not sure it made me feel better that he was making my service call a priority, but I knew that a woman alone like this is very vulnerable. I grew up in Manhattan and had learned my "street smarts" firsthand.

The dispatcher gave me the name of the towing service to expect and he told me not to accept help from anyone else. I couldn't understand the name he told me, so I asked him to spell it. I heard E-L and some other letters I wasn't sure of. Within ten minutes, Elite Towing drove up. The cavalry had arrived! Now I felt safe enough to get out of my car and see what the tire looked like. It was a mess of mangled rubber, pretty much what I had expected from the sound of it. As bad as it looked, only the tire and rim were damaged. They put the spare tire on and told me I could drive on it.

I called NYU again and was told I could still come in. They would be able to do at least some of the evaluation. I had gotten this far, so

I figured I might as well keep going, even though my body had yet to calm down. The evaluation, which had been so elevated in my mind, seemed inconsequential now. I had just driven four miles, monitoring the status of my blown-out tire by its sound, and resolved the situation using my cell phone—under stress. What more was an evaluation going to tell me?

It seems almost trivial to discuss this now, but the evaluation showed that my new ear was doing quite nicely. I could understand sentences at just about 100 percent. With single syllable words, it scored 66 percent. My other ear scored 74 percent, which is in the range it had always been. But with both ears listening together, I was able to repeat 82 percent of the single syllable words. That was the good news. The flip side was that testing in noise didn't show any advantage of both ears listening together. I wasn't that surprised, because in this test the noise was coming out of the same speaker as the test sentences. It's usually when noise is coming from different locations that I seem to be able to function better with two ears. There was no time left to do other noise evaluations, so I don't know how I would have fared under other test conditions.

With all this commotion, I haven't even talked about the mapping session I had two days prior. The mapping protocols are so routine and simple with these new processors, it was practically a nonevent. This time, however, I did notice that each ear heard the mapping tones differently. The new ear didn't perceive the lowest tones as deeply as the old ear could. There's no way to know, at this point in time, if they will eventually equalize.

The auditory therapy session this time focused on single syllable words. We went through some flash cards with paired words, the kind I was having trouble with. We then discussed some of the websites that have good practice resources—either word lists, sentences, or passages. We also discussed what I had been doing for practice, and once again my choices were right on target. They included phone practice, single word exercises, and recorded passages. We decided that there was no need for me to keep coming back for more sessions, so I will continue on my own, at my own pace and discretion.

The last appointment this week, with my surgeon, was just to make sure I was healing up well. He felt the various bumps along my scalp and examined the surgical site. I have to laugh because that reminded me of the nineteenth century pseudoscience, phrenology, which claimed that personality traits could be discerned by the bumps on one's head. That theory has long since been discredited, but there's an intriguing relevance. My CI experiences continue to reveal intriguing facets of my own personality.

DECEMBER 22, 2008 Small Surprises

The calendar keeps marching along, and the carefully laid plans for surgery dates, activations, mappings, evaluations, and surgical check-ups have all been accomplished—right on target. The main goal, actually, had been to finish all these tasks and get down to Florida before the northern winter weather hit in full force. We started driving last week, took a few days to visit family and go sightseeing, and arrived at our destination right on schedule. Also, as if on schedule, two snowstorms pummeled New Jersey three days after we left.

The last time we did this New Jersey/Florida car trip, in March, it was in reverse and in silence after my cochlear implant stopped working. We had to head back north then for the revision surgery that would allow me to hear once again. I knew full well that the drive this time—with sound—would be full of compare-and-contrast opportunities to discuss. It was so obvious—of course it was going to be better to hear than to travel in silence. And of course it was almost inevitable that I was going to have experiences of hearing better with two ears.

Surprisingly, though, driving in silence and driving with two functioning ears wasn't all that different for me. I enjoy crossword and Sudoku puzzles, which eat up boring travel time, and my husband enjoys listening to the radio and CDs. We were never going to chat nonstop for hours on end, anyway, so as long as I was the passenger, riding in silence or not didn't seem to make that much difference. Not blatantly, anyway.

I had another little surprise, even though I figured something like this would happen eventually during the trip. I was completely absorbed in my puzzles when I began to realize that I was also hearing and understanding the lyrics of the CD playing—Allan Sherman's Jewish humor song parodies. I guess with two ears, my brain can multitask! Some of these songs are almost classic, so I knew them from my youth, but there were others I hadn't heard before. Humor like this typically relies on puns, sound-alike words, and unexpected references. Precisely what makes it so funny also makes it difficult to hear correctly because context doesn't help—and this material really packed a punch. Every word, every phrase was carefully crafted and quickly delivered. For me, it was almost magical—as if someone had suddenly activated the switch that turned on the words. Some songs were more difficult than others, but this was new to me. To be able to hear those half-sung/half-spoken lyrics that fast and so well? Score another one for two ears!

Now comes the part of the trip I hadn't expected at all. Whenever we hit a bump in the road or a pothole or some rough terrain, my brain went into a mini-frenzy. "Arlene, the tire is making noise again! Listen to the tires—are we in trouble again?!" Oh, swell! My stressful tire experience the week before has left me with my very first bilateral auditory memory—the raucous sound of a blown-out tire as it's going flat while being driven for miles on its rim. Now it seems that any unusual tire sounds trigger a traumatic response of anxiety and primeval fear. Score another one for two ears!

Thankfully, this recent car crisis was only the second time in almost forty years of driving that I ever had trouble on the road. I remember all too well, though, the first time I had to summon AAA road service—eleven years ago, when my hearing was at its worst—six months before getting my first cochlear implant. The circumstances surrounding that experience were a little strange, and in stark contrast to this last episode.

I was driving a Saab 9000 Turbo back then. I loved that car because the turbo engine made me feel incredibly empowered. It was a great feeling, considering that my hearing was so poor I couldn't even listen to the radio. Unfortunately, that supercharged engine began to overheat, not in the wilds of upper Manhattan like last week, but on 54th Street just off Fifth Avenue. For a bad situation, it was the perfect location—next to the Museum of Modern Art and in front of the historic University Club townhouse, probably one of the safest places to land a turbo engine. The smoke was cascading from under the hood. I have no idea if it made any noise. Before I could panic, a woman appeared at my window with a cell phone in hand, asking if I needed help. Then the doorman from the University Club came down to assist as well. The woman called AAA, and the doorman directed traffic as the tow truck came to take me back to New Jersey. After that experience, we ended up trading in my "muscle" car for one with a better reliability rating.

I know people have differing interpretations of life's happenings, but the parameters of that car crisis have always seemed a little curious to me. Breaking down at a most fortuitous location and having what I have to describe as angels appearing on cue—it still gives me pause. Contrast that with my latest car crisis—being caught in an area where I couldn't even stop or get out of my car, and having to drive precariously for miles, with no angels in sight. But on more careful consideration, being equipped with two ears and a cell phone, I already possessed all the help I needed, didn't I? My only battle scar was the auditory memory of the experience, which pales in comparison to the emotional trauma of navigating life's challenges while deaf.

The last little surprise of my journey south happened while lighting the Chanukah candles this evening. I've been singing those ritual blessings for decades, but as soon as I began this time, my eyes lit up. I could hear my own voice with both ears, and the melody suddenly sounded new, ethereal, and—well—pretty. I had never heard myself like that before. It was almost as if I were listening to someone else. It's bewildering to think that my own voice had been hidden within me all these years, or that a second ear could make such a difference. I could go on to describe how Chanukah is about miracles, but it's enough to say that even small surprises can touch our hearts with wonder.

JANUARY 3, 2009 Matched Marvels

I'm starting to wonder when having two ears will begin to feel routine and "ho-hum." Not yet—not even after three months. Wearing these matched marvels behind my ears still makes me feel superpowered. And why shouldn't it? If you could suddenly do things you hadn't done in decades, you'd feel superpowered, too!

I guess what's feeding these feelings are my experiences with the end-of-year celebrations—so much noise, yet so much hearing! New Year's Eve was spent in a Brazilian restaurant at a table for six, with live entertainment. I only imbibed champagne at midnight, so my recollections are clear. My hearing was not the focus of the evening. That's an interesting way of putting it, but accurate. As anyone with a hearing loss knows, if you can escape thinking about your hearing, that is a major triumph, indeed!

The evening before, at a dinner for four with my daughter and her husband, the situation was similar—with a twist. The tables were more spread out, but the background conversation was very loud. My daughter said she was having trouble in this environment. I was not. *Hmmm?* Even people with normal hearing have to concentrate more when there's a lot of background noise—nothing unusual about that. But what is interesting is that in certain noisy situations, my processors pull in the closest speech sounds above the background noise and make it seem as though I'm in a "hearing bubble" with the people at my table. Superpowers indeed! Yes, granted, my lipreading skills probably helped, and this bubble only seems to happen in certain noisy situations, but it was definitely happening this time!

What's perplexing, though, is how to quantify this on hearing tests. I just received the written report of my hearing evaluation done three weeks ago, and there was no obvious evidence of "matched marvel superpowers." Two ears did seem to function better than one, but on the only noise test we had time for that day, I did not do better with two ears. Not all noisy environments are the same, of course, and a soundproof booth is not real life. The tests did show that my older ear alone, now using its new processor for nine months, had improved at listening in noise. It's likely that my newer ear will also score better as time goes on, and both ears together as well.

That said, I remember being frustrated with the test itself. It didn't seem to take into consideration some of the realities of a novice bilateral implant user. For example, the tests were given one after the other, which is a distinct disadvantage when testing the new ear. It takes a few minutes for my brain to refocus on the new ear after listening with the older ear alone or both together. There were some practice words built into the test, but I still felt that wasn't enough for my brain to make the transition. I don't even know if this had any impact on the results, but it left me feeling frustrated. I wanted to say, "Hey, wait, wait! This ear's not ready to listen yet!" But time was of the essence, so the test rolled on.

The single syllable word tests, which are hard because there are no contextual clues, also had me thinking. I know from the practice I've been doing that I sometimes miss the word on the first try, but get it when it is repeated. Somehow my brain is not always able to process the word entirely the first time, but has enough information to get it right the second time. The test scores only reflect whether I can repeat the word after hearing it once. Maybe data related to hearing a word on two tries is not important, but there's a psychological element at play here as well. Saying those words a second time could increase the probability of getting the word right and feeling good about it. Considering how much emotional baggage people with hearing loss bring into testing booths, I'm sure I'm not the only person who would welcome anything that tilts the odds toward having a more pleasant experience in those cubicles.

For the twenty-five years I was losing my hearing, every trip into a testing booth was depressingly negative since the test results were always worse, worse, worse. Only when I got my first CI did I begin to see these cubicles in a more positive light. I'm not surprised to discover that I still harbor intense emotions about hearing evaluations. I'm sure I'm not unique.

Outside the testing booths, in the real world, I've discovered that my eavesdropping capabilities are improving! I never paid much attention to other people's conversations because, unless I was staring, they were essentially out of range. Now I'm finding their words and phrases filtering into my subconscious. This is new to me. I hadn't really anticipated this as a category of bilateral hearing. It must be part of the superpower package, I guess. With all the cell phone conversations whirling around me, I'll definitely keep an ear (or two) to the ground!

JANUARY 11, 2009 One Good Turn

I turned to my name yesterday.

I've been waiting for this moment for a while now—three months and one week, to be exact. I had been getting some nibbles, but nothing I could definitively put the label *directionality* on. It snuck up on me—I didn't have to try or even think about it. It just happened.

We're in Florida now, so instead of shoveling and shivering, we were sauntering through an outdoor antique show with sunhats and sunglasses on. We struck our usual pace—sometimes I walk ahead of Ira, sometimes behind. Out of the sunny blue, I heard my name, and without a moment's hesitation, I spun around and saw Ira walking toward me from about twenty feet away. We both looked at each other, knowing full well what had just happened. I had not only heard him from that distance, but I had turned in the direction of his voice. That was the first time in decades that I had been able to do that.

When I first got my CI eleven years ago, I remember the thrill of being able to hear my own name. I no longer had to be tapped, touched, or jabbed to get my attention. My name was the useful communication tool it was meant to be. The reality, though, was that with one ear, I had no idea where a sound was coming from. If Ira called my name from a distance, I would invariably look upward, even though, intellectually, I knew that didn't make any sense at all! My brain was trying its best but didn't have enough information, so Ira would usually provide it. "Turn around," or, "Look to your left," he would direct. It was almost a game. Sort of funny, but I'm still surprised I kept my sense of humor about it. I guess I didn't get upset because I was still so thankful to hear my name at all.

But now, without any prompting, to turn to my name? With no instructions on where to look? That was the elusive bilateral advantage that I was told would take some time to develop. It's still a little new, so I wonder if I will miss the "Where Are You?" game. Not likely. This milestone brings me one step closer to that ever-elusive "normal hearing."

This epiphany wasn't totally unexpected. I did have those "nibbles" this past week that I would describe as *directionality lite*— not quite decisive signals, but a sense that I wasn't lost in space, either. The first inkling came when I was taking a walk and heard someone say, "beep-beep." I somehow instinctively looked over my right shoulder, and there was a man on a bicycle right behind me! I stepped to my left as he rode past me and said, "Thank you." It all happened so quickly, and with such grace—a virtual directionality dance, choreographed for two ears and a bicycle! It was what people with normal hearing would do without giving it a second thought. That is the confounding nature of hearing loss—such monumental efforts and equipment needed to do the mundane.

The next nibble came on a walk through a wetlands bird sanctuary, one we had visited several times before. Listening to birdcalls is nothing new to me. The new processors bring in these sounds so much clearer than my old processor did. I can even identify some birds by their sounds and songs—pretty impressive! This week, though, something was different. I was starting to sense what direction the birdcalls were coming from. Again, this wasn't quite directionality because I wasn't really sure. But Ira verified whether my perceptions were correct, and incredibly, they almost always were. No matter what the birdcall—coots, anhingas, moorhens, purple gallinules, red-wing blackbirds—I was able to guess (I wasn't sure) their direction.

To be honest, I'm also not exactly sure how purple gallinules sound, but I do love the way it feels to say that name out loud! I have other favorite bird names as well. Try saying *roseate spoonbill*! That has to be a speech pathologist's delight—a veritable smorgasbord of mouth movements in one species! And for my encore—try *limpkin*, a rare mottled-brown bird that I can actually identify by squawk. It's not just serendipity that's driving me to mention these names. I'm hearing my own voice more clearly now and that seems to make my mouth and tongue want to move with more precision. I guess in addition to directionality, my speech articulation is being bumped up a notch as well.

Getting back to the birds—as we were coming into the home-stretch of this mile-around boardwalk, I heard another call—a *toot-toot* that sounded more like a construction vehicle backing up than a bird, and it was coming from the direction of the road, about three-quarters of a mile away. I asked Ira if he heard it, too, and—I still can't believe this—he verified that it was, indeed, a construction vehicle! I was so proud. I even got the trick question right! This had to be the most glorious hearing evaluation I've ever experienced, done in the most exquisite of locations—Mother Nature's testing booth!

I'm trying to decide whether the practice I've been doing with my new ear has anything to do with the directionality I'm now experiencing or whether this would be happening anyway. I don't know if there's a way to tell, but it certainly couldn't have hurt! Aside from daily phone call practice with each ear, I've continued to work on single syllable words with my new ear. I've decided to keep track of the words I miss and I discovered that most of my errors are with the *T* and *K* sounds. No matter how many times I repeat certain words, they still don't sound right. The word *tape*, for example, sounds like *cape* to me, even though I can hear the word *cape* correctly. Context would probably take care of this in real life, but continued practice will likely resolve this problem, too.

I've also discovered that my two ears are usually working in tandem, as my directionality experiences have shown. With music and general comprehension, it doesn't seem to matter that my new ear alone isn't as strong as the old one. My brain merges them, and even the sound is becoming more blended. That little echo effect isn't always apparent now. I know that somehow it must be beneficial to continue working on strengthening the new ear, even though I can't say for sure that it helps when using both ears together.

I had one curious experience this week where the two ears were *not* functioning in tandem, and this little revelation caught me by surprise. I was sitting on the terrace of my seventh-floor apartment, overlooking the treetops, when a screeching bird flew by. I love these face-to-face encounters! At the very moment of the screech, I experienced the compression effect in my new ear—the result of the automatic gain control (AGC) software feature that dims loud sounds automatically. But my old ear didn't blink. It had no apparent muting or compression effect from that bird screech. Why the difference in responses? The answer was most likely the length of time using CI processors, and specifically, the amount of experience using AGC software.

Hallelujah! I finally have the opportunity to tell the bizarre little tale that introduced me to the concept of AGC software. Back in 2001, when I upgraded from a body-worn processor to a behind-the-ear model, I upgraded the software I was using as well. The new software had a more advanced version of AGC, but I was cautioned that adapting to it would be challenging. It seems that since my brain had already adapted to a different version, it would have more trouble with the new program than if I had used it from the beginning. I wasn't deterred, so I asked to try it out. After just a few sentences with this new AGC setting, the sounds were cutting in and out, making the program virtually unusable. I wasn't about to give up, though, so I asked to keep this setting on one of my programs and I'd play with it during the week.

Each day I would switch to the program with the new AGC setting, using it for longer periods each time. By the end of the week, I had no trouble using that program all the time. Normal conversations sounded natural and only very loud sounds, like pots clanging, would cause that muted, cutting-out response.

This is really so bizarre. Nothing had changed in the course of that week other than my brain's perception of the sound it was receiving. I truly would not have believed this was possible if I hadn't experienced it myself. What was, essentially, a totally unusable program at the beginning of the week—cutting out at normal conversation levels—had morphed into a program that was not only totally usable, but now also had features to respond to loud sounds in a way that simulated the way a normal ear functions. That's how it was explained to me—that somewhere in our development, the human ear does filter out loud sounds to some extent. It is such a natural process that no one notices it. And that's what was happening with my adaptation to this AGC software—a gradual change of perception so that I no longer noticed when it was kicking in, except with very loud sounds. The adaptation to this software didn't stop after one week, though. It continued for years, to the extent that now I rarely notice any dimming of sound at all.

And that brings us to the situation on the terrace with the screeching bird. My old ear is literally the "old pro" at this—it can handle sudden noise. The new ear is still learning. Evidently, the brain controls this perception of loud sounds in each ear separately. It's not one of those merged functions, like music, directionality, or functioning in noise. This is a fascinating little revelation, but the important headline this week is still the one about directionality:

ARLENE TURNED TO HER NAME!

JANUARY 16, 2009 Orientation

It turns out that last week's breakthrough—turning to my name—was not a fluke. Ira keeps calling me, and I keep turning around! My personal best so far is being called from about seventy-five feet away. This is directionality for sure! At first, this seemed like a new toy, but now I'm finding it very useful. It's adding a dynamic that I hadn't even realized was missing.

If I can respond to being called from a distance, that means I'm connected to people by voice alone. Did you want to show me something interesting or tell me something "of the moment"? I'm available —just call my name and if I'm within earshot, I'll look your way. Ira called me from seventy-five feet away because he wanted to show me something. Walking to get me was simply not practical for something not terribly important. I now wonder how many times I was left out of the little stuff just because I wouldn't have turned around.

This gives additional meaning to the term *directionality*. It is not simply the ability to tell where a sound is coming from. It is also being able to orient yourself to your surroundings by sound—a much broader and more inclusive concept.

I'm starting to notice this more as I go about routine tasks. Just yesterday, I was paying for a purchase at a drug store counter. The cashier was robotically going through her paces—no chitchat, all business. I handed her cash, expecting her to give me change, but she wasn't even making eye contact with me. Then I heard *ka-ching-a-ching*, the sound of change dropping down a chute somewhere to my right. And there they were—the coins were waiting for me in a place I hadn't expected, not near the cash register at all, but three feet over beyond the bagging area. The cashier never looked at me. She assumed, of course, that I would hear the money and take it. I did.

Imagine the scenario, though, with one ear. I probably would have heard the coins dropping and looked all around me—maybe finding them without help, maybe not. If I had no hearing at all, I wouldn't even have had a chance. Once again, two ears, working as designed, had me oriented to my surroundings by sound. And in the process, allowed me to do a mundane task, just like everybody else.

It's interesting that this ability to localize sound is kicking in at three and a half months. That time frame has special significance for me. We took my son, Michael, to have his hearing tested when he was three months old. It was recommended because I had a hearing loss, so he was considered at higher risk. We had intended to have his hearing tested in the hospital when he was born, but his forceps delivery was so difficult, and I was such a mess, that we opted to wait. We took him to the League for the Hard of Hearing (now called the Center for Hearing and Communication), where an audiologist who was an expert in infant testing evaluated him. As we watched, though, our hearts sank. Michael didn't seem to respond to any of the sounds. When the test was complete, we were preparing for the worst, so we were absolutely astonished when the audiologist came out and reported that she wished she'd had a video camera. Michael had shown the perfect responses for a three-month-old! *How could that be?*, we thought. He hadn't moved. And then we learned that three-month-olds don't turn to sound! His responses were subtle—changes in breathing, eye movement, sucking—all showing he was hearing. Normal!

Now I'm the one learning to turn to sound at three and a half months, with the first breakthrough responding to my husband's voice. It makes me wonder whether Michael would have turned to my voice in that testing booth thirty-four years ago. My hunch is that he would have.

I'm beginning to build on this skill—as that drug store cashier experience shows—reacting to more sounds and the direction they're coming from. I did a little checking, and it seems that, on average, babies start turning to sound at five months of age. At three and a half months, that makes me one very precocious infant.

JANUARY 19, 2009 Born Yesterday

I keep thinking about my revised definition of directionality: being able to orient yourself to your surroundings by sound. My mind conjures up this image of a site map of sounds, with me in the center. That is the exact same imagery I described in my Thanksgiving episode two months ago when I did so well in noise. I was able to separate out the different conversations and even background noise then, but I couldn't yet shut my eyes and distinguish the direction of those sounds. That experience was evidently the precursor to what's happening now—envisioning the same site map but relying less and less on visual cues to pinpoint the location of those sounds.

From this perspective, it's apparent that hearing better in noise and directionality aren't two discrete (ie, unconnected) abilities. They are evidently two different applications of binaural function, which rely on that site map concept. That site map didn't exist on day one of my bilateral hearing experience. It took me at least a month to develop the sound landscape perception that facilitated functioning in noise, and three and a half months to begin envisioning this landscape by sound alone, which is evidently the basis of directionality.

I was only half kidding about being a precocious infant, turning to sounds at three and a half months. I'm starting to suspect that all my hearing experiences may be related to infant hearing behaviors. For instance, I'm particularly curious about that happy feeling I sensed in my first two weeks of binaural hearing. My October 17 episode, entitled "Finding Happiness," described this feeling. I'm usually sensitive to nuances of mood, and now I'm not convinced that the happy mood I experienced was simply because it felt nice to hear with two ears—even considering the many benefits. I think it's more complex than that.

Consider my daughter, Emily, as a newborn. She was born ten days after her due date and actually smiled on her first day of life. I know they say that newborns can't smile, but there was no mistaking her open-mouthed, crooked little smile as one of real joy. I'm adept at nonverbal communication, as many people with hearing loss are, and I can read faces very well. To me, Emily's smile was saying, "I'm so happy to finally see you! I've been listening to your voice for months!" All newborns probably have some cerebral stimulation when hearing their mothers' voices for the first time, to facilitate bonding, but Emily's smile was the tip-off about a happiness factor.

The question is, was her smile the result of hearing and seeing me, or was her infant brain programmed to feel happy when she heard what would most likely be her mother's voice? Whichever it is, I sense that my own happy feelings when first hearing with two ears are somehow related to this newborn response. The gatekeeper in the brain that coordinates binaural hearing could easily flip on the *happy* switch when it is stimulated for the first time and for a few weeks afterward. This actually makes sense to me and correlates with my gut feeling that my brain was being tweaked to feel happy. Mother Nature apparently assumes that anyone new to binaural hearing must be a newborn and will be treated as such!

What else fits this paradigm? Newborns have a startle reflex to loud sounds, which gradually diminishes after five to six months, as the baby's hearing mechanism somehow adapts. This correlates with my adaptation to the AGC software, which controls sudden loud sounds. I've already described how adapting to this software is a "brain thing." Newborns most likely go through a similar process. I've determined that this is not a binaural function, though, as each ear seems to adapt separately.

There's one other behavior that seems to emulate a newborn trait. In my January 11 episode, I mentioned loving the way it felt to say words out loud. I also noted that hearing my own voice more clearly makes me want to move my mouth and tongue with more precision. In other words, I'm babbling! Babies start to babble at about three months of age. I'm right on target! I had a similar experience adapting to my single new processor last summer, except without that feeling of happiness. I assume the brain's gatekeeper for binaural hearing flipped the happy switch this time, to reinforce and encourage this babbling behavior. The operative question, of course, is, "When will I *stop* babbling!?" Not to worry—we'll know soon enough.

I am a little puzzled about all this. Evidently when I started hearing with two ears, I triggered an infant hearing launch sequence! First, the binaural coordinator in my brain flipped on a *feel happy* switch, which made me love hearing with two ears right from the start, forming a special bond with the first voices I heard. I immediately started adapting to the software that controls loud sounds, the CI counterpart to the startle reflex. By one month, I began to develop an ability to separate sounds, which facilitated hearing in noise. At three months, I started babbling, listening to my own voice and enjoying practicing more precise tongue and mouth movements. And at three and a half months, I started turning to sound, beginning with the voice I had bonded with in the first two weeks. Now, I am branching out to other sounds as well. Following this path, I figure that I will just get better at these skills with more time and practice.

What's particularly striking is that the sound delivered by the CI processors is of high enough quality to convince the brain that this is the real thing! And I'm still intrigued by my ability to turn to my husband's voice from a distance. But since his voice was the primary voice I bonded with those first two weeks, it makes sense that his would be the one I would turn to first, and also be able to identify from a larger radius. For an infant, that would be an important behavioral trait—to be able to zone in on its source of food, comfort, and safety. That brings to mind those penguin documentaries, which show the uncanny ability of baby penguins to find their mothers among thousands of identical-looking birds, by sound alone. Now it doesn't seem quite so bizarre. I could pick out my husband's voice at seventy-five feet without looking, and he only called my name once. I'm sure Mother Nature never intended for me to bond with my husband's voice, but then again, Mother Nature never imagined deaf people hearing, either.

As a baby with normal hearing, I actually did bond with my mother's voice. I know this because when my hearing was at its worst decades later, I was still able to hear and understand her voice, even when I couldn't hear most frequencies. The sad irony is that although she would have been the best person to repeat what others were saying to me, by that time her Alzheimer's made it difficult for her to do so. I won't even describe the many layers of sadness of that situation.

Now that I've explained my theories on this binaural hearing continuum, I realize that it doesn't really make much difference for me. I'm still going to practice listening, to optimize my hearing in real-life situations. It does seem particularly relevant, however, for infants and children with cochlear implants. If binaural hearing does trigger certain basic infant behaviors, particularly bonding with a caregiver, that is significant indeed.

FEBRUARY 1, 2009   The Sand and the Sea Reprise

One of my favorite activities is walking on the beach. There's a majestic serenity about it—the cascading waves with crests of white and shades of blue merging with the sky above, the feel of the sand shifting beneath the soles of my feet, and of course, the sounds. It was sadly silent last March when my processor stopped working and the sound of my world stopped abruptly. That didn't keep me from walking on the beach, but I was relieved to hear the ocean once again, last August, with my new processor. Since then, I have been looking forward to returning with two ears, anticipating an enchanting experience—surely something magical to relate.

My first walk on the beach several weeks ago, listening with two ears, sounded lovely. But when I checked the sound with one ear, it also sounded lovely. Listening with two ears sounded a little fuller, but nothing special enough to announce on these pages. The second walk on the beach a little later held a similar experience—and again, I can't say I was disappointed, but I was a little bewildered as to why two ears weren't having the impact I thought they would.

This week brought me to MacArthur Beach State Park, where the stretch of beach is left natural and undeveloped, the *real* Florida. The sand was strewn with seaweed, and the shoreline wasn't straight so the waves were more erratic. I started my walk and again tried listening with one ear alone and then both together. One ear alone was still beautiful—the roaring surf, the gusts of wind. Then I put the second ear on. It did sound fuller, but there was something about it that still eluded me.

I kept walking, and it was then that I recalled the note cards I had won as a door prize eleven years ago at a temple event—the ones with a nautilus shell on the front surrounded by the words LISTEN CLOSELY. There was always something a little strange about those note cards—just a little too perfect. I had always thought that message meant to look for deeper meaning in the ordinary events of life. Now, though, they seemed to be beckoning me to do exactly as stated: Listen closely, Arlene. I stopped and faced the ocean. I was now on a stretch of shoreline that was empty—the high-rise condominiums were a distant blur, and all the beach chairs and surfers were nowhere near. I was alone with the sand and the sea.

Yes, with two ears the sound was fuller, but this time, I had the feeling that I was in the center of a sound landscape, similar to what I described at Thanksgiving and with my first experiences with directionality. With one ear, I was simply an observer looking at beautiful scenery with the audio on. With two ears, I was experiencing a very sophisticated version of directionality. It wasn't just stereo. It was surround sound, and I was being drawn into this landscape, not as an observer but as a participant. It enveloped me, embraced me—two ears, at one with nature.

I even checked again, using one ear and then two, just to be sure. With two ears, there was a feeling of being connected to my surroundings—another triumph for assessing directionality in Mother Nature's testing booth. And my initial instinct about this simple beach walk was proven correct as well. Being enveloped by the sounds of the ocean was an enchanting experience. There is no doubt that Hannah Senesh, the poet of "Eli, Eli," had experienced the sand and the sea with two ears as well:

> I pray that these things never end,
> The sand and the sea,
> The rush of the water,
> The crash of the heavens,
> The prayer of my heart.

As I walked along the beach, my mind began to wander. That's why I love these strolls—the serenity of it all. My thoughts turned to the talk I was scheduled to give—the first time I would be discussing my device failure and the path that led to my binaural hearing. Perhaps I could find a spiral-shaped shell to use in my talk—not a perfect one, but one that was broken. As I had learned many years ago from my daughter Emily, broken spiral-shaped shells are the most exquisite treasures because they reveal a beauty inside that would never be seen if they were whole.

For the twenty-four days last March when I had no hearing, a broken spiral shell was the perfect symbol of my "broken CI world." The wisdom hidden within was that of a looking glass existence— everything was backward. The world was silent instead of noisy. Trying to function in the hearing world was futile, so withdrawing was the better option—the total opposite of the can-do spirit I had nurtured for decades. Now that I'm hearing with two ears, the message is more direct: A broken spiral shell, revealing intricate structures, is an apt reminder of the complex hidden mechanisms that are allowing me to hear.

As I walked a little farther, there it was, waiting for me: a spiral-shaped whelk, bigger than all the other shells on the beach. Perfectly broken, revealing its complex internal beauty: exactly what I was looking for. And that is what fascinates me—how nature's intricate design of coordinating two ears is working in tandem with my two cochlear implants—enabling a simple walk on the beach to become a majestic connection to nature.

FEBRUARY 16, 2009 The Visit

Did you ever have an experience so wonderful, so different, so exhilarating, and so intellectually challenging that you wondered if anything would ever compare to it again? I did—eight years ago.

I had been asked to participate in a panel presentation for the National Institutes of Health's (NIH) annual Neural Prosthesis Program conference, held at their facilities in Bethesda, Maryland. This annual gathering gave researchers who work on prosthetic devices that interface with the human nervous system the opportunity to share the progress of their grant projects with their colleagues. That year, 2001, someone had the excellent idea to invite users of neural prosthetic devices to describe their experiences. It seems that many of these researchers never get the chance to meet the people who use the devices they've helped develop.

I was delighted to receive the call to participate. I was paired with the former director of the NIH's Neural Prosthesis Program, who had been a leader in cochlear implant research and development. His task was to read through my book and act as facilitator during my portion of the panel presentation. The actual presentation was but one facet of this experience, though. I was literally thrown into a community of brilliant minds. "Working the hallways" took on new meaning with this group. It was thrilling to share ideas and experiences with this rarefied crowd. Going out to dinner with several of them—getting a glimpse into their world, especially their level of humor—was both insightful and delightful. After two days, we had definitely bonded, and they even persuaded me to do an

unofficial book signing. I was floating on air for days after that conference, with so many thoughts swirling through my mind. During
the ensuing months, and even years, I kept thinking those were the
two most enchanting days I had ever spent.

Just a few months ago, when planning a trip to California, I immediately thought to request a visit to Advanced Bionics's headquarters,
where my cochlear implants were made. Since I was in the process of
writing these chronicles, I figured it would be helpful to speak with
some of the tech people, audiologists, and others, to get additional
background and insights on current cochlear implant technology. I
also offered to speak to their staff members. I always enjoy talking
about my own cochlear implant experience—just put a microphone
in my hands, point me toward an audience, and let me loose!

My request to visit was graciously granted, and we worked out
a schedule that encompassed all my suggestions, including presentations to staff members. It turned out they have a "Connect to
Patient" program, which is designed to allow their staff members to
meet actual cochlear implant users. The rationale for this program
was almost identical to the one I participated in at the NIH conference—to meet real people whose lives are impacted by these devices.
That has to be both humbling and inspiring for an employee, no
matter what one's role in the cochlear implant process.

Now the cogs of my mind were in gear once again—the parameters of this visit were almost identical to my awesome NIH experience
eight years prior. Would this be—*could* this be—another wonderful,
different, exhilarating, intellectually challenging experience? It had
all the potential ingredients.

But first I had to get to California! Fortunately, we had a direct
flight into Los Angeles on JetBlue, the airline with the seatback televisions. This would be my first flight using two ears, but I didn't think
there was going to be much difference. I just love when my own
preconceived notions are so wrong!

What I hadn't counted on was that the wonderful benefit of
"surround sound" that comes with having two ears also applies to
airplane cabin noise! *Ahhh*—now I finally understand what everyone
complains about, and why headphone manufacturers have rushed to

develop noise-canceling products. With one CI, the cabin noise isn't particularly bad. It's just like the rushing waves of the ocean—you're an observer. But with two ears, it envelops you. Being enveloped by the sound of the ocean is fine—but cabin noise? Maddeningly annoying! I did want the normal hearing experience, so I stoically left both processors on and listened to the television through headphones, which diverted most of the noise. (On the late-night flight back east, I cheated and took off both processors and went to sleep—the advantages of being bionic!)

It took a lot of thought, but I finally laid out the plan for my presentations, using some of my writings, anecdotes, and even the broken spiral shell I had plucked from the beach two weeks before. My biggest concern, though, was my own voice. I had never given a presentation while listening with two ears. I wasn't sure how I would sound to myself or to others. I also was concerned about my emotional state, wondering if I could get through discussing my device failure and days of silence without bursting into tears.

My style is to be upfront about my concerns when speaking in public, so I let the audience know about the worries I had about my own voice. Just talking about that subject allowed me to do a voice assessment at the same time. My voice was good—I actually liked the way I sounded and I found myself enunciating very precisely. I got through the device failure and days of silence portions totally dry-eyed—actually, too dry-eyed. This was a little bizarre because in my mental preparations, I always ended up with tears in my eyes.

What was different? I was talking out loud. I was hearing my own voice with two ears. I was that precocious infant again—and I was babbling, listening to myself speak! Clinical babbling—which means Mother Nature gives the brain a *happy* tweak because it wants to encourage this verbal practice. And that's exactly how I felt—so happy to hear my own voice, and babbling to a very receptive audience! I truly wonder when this babbling phase will wear off—hopefully not soon. It's far too much fun doing public speaking this way!

Or another explanation for the lack of tears is that I disdain public displays of emotion. I happen to like the babbling theory better, and frankly, I think that's the correct one.

I also walked into that presentation with a confidence I hadn't felt before—a command and connection to my environment that is coming from my four months' experience hearing with two ears. I also knew that I would be able to field questions from a distance and just function *better*—and that translates to a reduction in stress and a calmer presence. I could actually feel it.

My next adventure was meeting with the tech people, something I was really looking forward to. In my life before children, back in the 1970s, I had been a systems programmer for New York Life Insurance Company. I wrote software in several languages, trained others, did troubleshooting, and wrote documentation, the descriptions of software systems. I was a real relic, though—I used keypunch cards, and the machines I worked on were dinosaurs.

My first stop was a session with programmers, getting a software tour. First they pulled up the fitting software, the computer program that the audiologist uses to map the cochlear implant. That was familiar to me, but I wanted to see the computer code—the actual programming instructions that produced this fitting software. They selected one programming routine that set up patient information. And there it was—exactly what I had wanted to see—actual computer language statements that I hadn't seen in thirty-five years! I saw the *if* and *then* instructions, and the memories came flooding back!

They explained that when they worked on a program, they took it out like a library book. That sounded familiar, too! I had worked on a library management system in my programming days, and it had the same goal: managing all the programs in the computer system. I had also written the documentation for the system, which was geared for both tech people and non-tech senior management. I received the highest accolade from one of the VPs, who told me, "This is the most understandable piece of writing that has ever come out of this insurance company!" This bodes well for what I'm about to describe.

Our next stop was to visit a programmer who was working on the software for the processor itself. These programs were written in assembly language, more appropriate for this application because it is closer to machine code, so it's more efficient and takes up less storage space. As soon as they pulled up the programming code, more memories came flooding back. We started talking about the "registers," and I blurted out, "Did you initialize the registers?" And we all laughed. I hadn't heard that term, which refers to how data is stored in a computer's memory, in thirty-five years! I was assured that they had, indeed, initialized the registers. The basics of programming were still the same—moving pieces of data from one location to another based on specific criteria. No magic—just logic.

But I still needed to know how the program on the computer screen got into my processor to make me hear. They explained that when the audiologist is finished with the mapping session, she then downloads the resulting program into my processor. The processor is a computer, and when the battery connection is made, the computer starts running the program. I asked if that was the same as *booting up the system*, which is what happens when you turn a computer on—and the answer was yes. The last computer I had programmed took up an entire floor at 28th Street and Madison Avenue, and it had special air conditioning, raised floors to accommodate the electrical cables, and ran the software by using a keypunch card reader. The computers allowing me to hear are sitting behind my ears. Astounding!

This tech tour was exactly what I had imagined and hoped it would be. We were all speaking the same language! They told me how happy they were that their technical work was helping people to hear. I understood, probably in greater depth than anyone, just what they meant. When I worked as a programmer, all my efforts went to improve the bottom line of an insurance company. When I left, I had no desire to go back because it was just too *sterile*, as I put it then. I couldn't have imagined back then—actually, no one could have imagined back then—the computer programming reality I'm living today.

My two-day adventure also included speaking casually to people in all areas of the company. One young woman told me that she had enjoyed hearing my presentation because my descriptions of living in silence helped her envision "walking in my footsteps." A young man told me the comparisons of my hearing to infant hearing behavior had struck a chord because he had an infant at home. I found my-self listening in a relaxed manner. That worrisome "which side are they on" behavior seems to have finally left, and with it has come a subtle change in the dynamics of my conversations. I'm listening more and that means people are telling me more. I like that. I learn more that way.

In many respects, this two-day visit was as wonderful, different, exhilarating and intellectually challenging as my NIH experience eight years ago. It, too, left me floating on air with many thoughts swirling through my mind. I definitely recommend having a once-in-a-lifetime adventure every few years.

FEBRUARY 23, 2009 Directionality Redux

Turning to the source of sound—that's directionality. It seems so simple in theory. Even quantifying it with hearing evaluations in a testing booth makes it appear so matter-of-fact. It's not. In fact, it's yet another example where the reality of hearing—actually living it—is so far removed from the testing booth, that I sometimes feel like stomping my feet with frustration! What happened?

My brain continues to develop and respond to binaural sound, that's what!

At three and a half months, I started turning to my husband's voice when he called my name. That replaced the exasperating "Where are you?" befuddlement I had endured with one ear. Now, at four and a half months, turning to Ira's voice has become a very reliable skill, and he finds that he can call me from any reasonable distance and I'll always turn around. That happened just the other day, in Costco, the cavernous warehouse store. We were both forag-ing for smoked salmon and decided to split up to speed the search. We ended up in different aisles, and then I heard, "ARLENE!" That made me turn instantly to Ira's voice. He was at least twenty-five feet away and he had a big smile on his face. One would think that after a month, this behavior would become somewhat routine, but it hasn't. It's not hard to figure out the reason. In this quest for hearing, we always seem to gloss over the impact of hearing loss on the people closest to us.

You don't wipe out in one month more than twenty-five years of not being able to get your wife's attention. I can read faces—and I can also read smiles—and I sensed there was more to Ira's smile than just his happiness at having me respond instantly to his call. So I asked, and I learned that when I had only one CI, he didn't always call my name, even though he knew that he could first get my attention and then give me clues to his precise location. Why not? It seems that my response was so bizarre—looking skyward and playing twenty questions—that he didn't want to embarrass me in certain social situations. He had taken on the burden and the stress of deciding when and where to call out my name in public. It crossed my mind that perhaps he was the one embarrassed by my "Where are you?" one-sided behavior, but after almost thirty-nine years of marriage, I know this is not the case. At our wedding, our first dance was "Someone to Watch Over Me"—and he does.

My thoughts, though, turn to children with CIs in the classroom and the school yard. Their classmates have no commitment to being sensitive or considerate of behaviors that aren't quite normal. Who watches over them? That also makes me think of the greater ease I'm having with casual conversations, no longer worrying about which side people are on. Put these two benefits of binaural hearing together, and the outcome is better socialization—something I *know* I'm doing better now—and I didn't have to learn it, having grown up with normal hearing. Children with hearing loss are at a much greater disadvantage when it comes to learning the subtle cues that are the building blocks of appropriate social behavior. Anything that gets them closer to normal interaction will most likely improve their socialization skills, something that is enormously important in every aspect of daily living.

But there's more to this issue of directionality.

I had lunch with two friends, one a hearing aid user and one a CI user. We have known each other for twenty years and, collectively, probably understand more about the nuances of hearing loss than any three people around. Ruth noticed immediately how relaxed I was. She could see it in my face. This was the first time we had spoken with each other since I acquired my second CI. She told me to compare pictures "before and after" going bilateral, and she was sure I'd be able to see a difference. We were engrossed in this discussion when I heard my name being called from the kitchen. I looked up and saw Charlotte smiling at me. She knew. We all knew that I never would have turned to my name like this with just one ear.

That marked the breakthrough that my directionality skills have expanded to other voices, not just my husband's. At four and a half months, this precocious infant is now able to turn to random voices!

But there's more.

I was taking one of my nature/listening/exercise walks. With my first CI, I listened to books on tape for practice while walking. Now I like to listen to the world around me with two ears. I consider that practice, too! The landscape in Florida is so beautiful—birds, flowers, sun, and sky. I'm often mesmerized by it all, and become absorbed in my own thoughts.

On this walk, I had literally hit my stride, turning the bend by the waterway that is a haven for waterfowl, when I heard, *SQUAWK!* Without a moment's hesitation, I whirled around and found myself staring eye-to-eye with a limpkin, a mottled-brown mini version of a flamingo. (For the full thousand-word imagery of this bird, I suggest doing an Internet image search.) My response was not discretionary—there was absolutely no thinking involved. Frankly, I was very surprised at how fast I reacted. It is not hard to figure out what had just happened here, either. We are wired and programmed to be alert to danger, a safety feature built into Mother Nature's original design. My autopilot pirouette was a reflexive response, and signaled that my binaural safety alerter was now enabled!

Safety—it's not a word that I had associated with directionality. But now that I have personally experienced this very basic protective behavior—instinctively turning to potential danger—you can understand why I want to rant and rave about it! Directionality isn't just a benign little behavioral nicety that makes life more convenient. It is the basis for both safety and socialization—two critical human behavioral skills. Whether it can be replicated in a testing booth is almost moot. As these behaviors become more natural to me with time and experience, I am even more in awe realizing how much I had been missing with only one ear.

MARCH 3, 2009 Hidden Agendas

I've continued to be fairly diligent about practicing my listening skills. I've continued to use my new ear alone for at least an hour each day. I still do single syllable word practice on my computer and phone practice with each ear. The goal has been to build up the new ear and eventually have it blend with the old. That seems a little simplistic now, considering all the recent hoopla over directionality, but it still is the basic objective. Does all this practice actually help? The short answer is yes—probably.

After five months, I can tell that I'm doing better with single syllable words. When I first started, I had to repeat the words over and over to get them to sound right. Now I can hear most of them correctly on the first try. That in itself is significant because I had experienced similar problems when I used hearing aids—I felt the need to have words repeated for my brain to process them. The benefits of this regimen have also carried over into real-life situations. Words like *coot* or *soap*, used in context, are now familiar to me, and I recognize them as words I've practiced. I also sense that these drills have strengthened the other speech sounds as well. But these "testing booth drills" only result in a "number of words correct" score. How this impacts practical life is where the true importance lies.

Having my new ear function better seems to be helping me field voices more reliably, enhancing casual conversation. This means I am more aware of my surroundings and able to respond more quickly, even without visual cues. I may even overhear something and comment on it. This is producing a subtle change in my behavior and—I'm a little hesitant to write this—even my personality. People seem to be responding to me a little differently—with more interest, more give-and-take. There must be some subtle timing cues at play here, some split-second communication signals that lie in the subconscious. If I have no hesitation at all in my responses, does that convey greater interest, greater sincerity? I think so.

At five months, I'm also finding that my hearing has not stabilized fully yet. Some days I need to put the volume up on my processors, and some days I need to put the volume down. My old ear seems to be rebelling, occasionally taking on a hazy quality. This is similar to its bouts with hoarseness that it typically developed when it was working on something new.

The old ear is still the dominant one. If I take the processor off the new ear, the world still sounds mostly the same. If I take the processor off the old ear, the new ear alone still sounds much more electronic. This is a little perplexing because the new ear does sound pretty normal in the morning when I use it alone—certainly good enough for me to use all day if I had to, although I don't. It must be similar to having something taste sour after eating something very sweet. The brain's perception gets skewed temporarily.

There have been some subtle shifts, though. I was talking on the phone using my old ear when the battery on the processor of my new ear died. The only thing that had changed was how I was hearing my own voice, but it sounded strange to me, which is an interesting development. That means I've gotten used to the sound of my own voice using two ears. This may not seem like much of a breakthrough, but it means the sound of two ears working together has evidently become the norm for my brain.

Something similar happened just a few days ago. After writing about "Someone to Watch Over Me" in a recent episode, I couldn't seem to get that tune out of my head. I finally ended up singing it out loud. I don't even know all the words and substituted "la-la-la" for the ones I couldn't remember. As I started singing, I stopped in my tracks. It was my mother singing—there was no mistaking the lilting tones and joyful demeanor. She used to sing to herself exactly that way—even using "la-la-las" for the words she didn't know. And the voice was hers as well. The question is—why is this coming up now? It took a little sleuthing, but I discovered that when I listen to myself sing using only my new ear, my voice sounds just like my mother's. When I listen with both ears, it is also the dominant sound, the first time that has ever happened.

All these shifts in perception must somehow be related to my practice regimen, though it is also possible that I would have reached this point anyway. There is no way to know for sure. I also have to laugh at how naive my original practice goals seem now. I couldn't possibly have known that "building up the new ear and having it blend with the old" would also evolve into becoming a more engaging conversationalist or discovering my mother's voice within my own.

APRIL 4, 2009 Tears of Joy

At six months, I can't say that having two ears has become routine yet, but the novelty is starting to wear off a bit. New listening environments still intrigue me, though, so I continue to test my ears "left, right, and together." It is still amazing to me that what seems so simple—listening with two ears—can sometimes be so complex.

This was demonstrated to me yet again as we started our spring migration back to New Jersey. We stopped at a gem of an attraction along the way: Bok Tower Gardens in Lake Wales, Florida—a National Historic Site that features a 205-foot art deco carillon tower situated amid lush gardens.

When we arrived, we were delighted to learn that a live concert was about to begin! We were seated in a beautifully landscaped area at the base of the tower, in view of a live video monitor showing the carillonneur perched at his keyboard high above us inside the tower. This sixty-bell carillon was played like an organ, pressing large keys with the hands and using the feet for the pedals that controlled the largest bells. It was fascinating watching how the melodies and harmonies were literally "hammered out," and I was very happy to be able to hear the clear tones of the chimes so well.

After the concert, the carillonneur came down for a question-and-answer session with his audience. This was such a treat! I knew absolutely nothing about carillons. As I followed the give-and-take of the discussion, I asked him if it was very loud playing up in the tower, so close to the bells. He looked squarely at me and replied, "What?" I repeated my question, and again he responded, "What?" On the third try, he laughed, shook my hand, and thanked me for being such a good sport. He had been pretending to have a hearing loss! He said someone always asks him that question. I could tell he had no inkling about my hearing loss, and I didn't say a word about it. I was very content to skip the entire subject.

We continued exploring the grounds, meandering through the manicured gardens. As we made our way along the labyrinth of pathways, the carillon began playing again, this time a recorded rendition of "America the Beautiful." We moved a little closer to the tower, stopping in front of a secluded lagoon beneath a canopy of treetops, surrounded by cascades of exotic flowers. The mission of the landscape designer had been to create a garden that would "touch the soul with its beauty," and this setting achieved its goal exquisitely.

The sound of the carillon was now so powerful, I had to know how it would sound with each ear separately and then together. First, I listened with the old ear. It heard the chimes beautifully. Then the new ear. It could hear the bell tones, but couldn't handle the complex harmonies clearly.

And finally, together. I burst into tears.

It was almost as if my brain didn't know what to do with the intensity of the sound or the setting. It was all too perfect, too magnificent. My head was being filled with the brilliance of the bells and their intricate harmonies, and my immediate reaction was euphoria. I was overwhelmed to the point of tears. The idyllic setting and my familiarity with this majestic song surely added to the experience.

The question still remains, though, how could listening with two ears make such a difference? I had just learned that carillon bells continue to resonate long after they are struck, unlike pianos or organs, so the intensity of sound builds with the harmony. Both of my CI processors must have been handling the complexities of these acoustics impeccably well. Each one was designed to separate the voices and process complex harmonies, but something else was happening when both ears were combined. Somehow, the area of my brain that coordinates two ears could interpret the signals it was receiving and envelop me with sound—powerfully so! It didn't matter that the signals were digital replicas. My brain knew just what to do with them. It also seemed able to activate the *happy* area of my brain, and it evidently sent a thunderbolt!

Even days later, I'm still thinking this over, amazed that listening with two ears could have such an enormous impact on my emotions.

APRIL 26, 2009 Lasting Impressions

I had always likened the cochlear implant adaptation process to creating a masterpiece. Adding the nuances and clarity of sound to a blank canvas was like filling in the background and shading of a fine painting. I even had a specific work in mind, Rembrandt's *Aristotle Contemplating a Bust of Homer*. The lighting, detail, sophisticated subject, composition, and even its lofty size epitomized the masterpiece I envisioned.

With my first CI, there was no question that the sounds and improved level of functioning they brought were a masterpiece in their own right. Even so, I was still seeking a degree of perfection that I now know was just not possible with that processor. There were limitations to what I could create using essentially one older paint box with a limited range of colors. My world of sound was surely magnificent compared to the blank canvas of deafness, but it was still only an approximation of the masterpiece I had in mind.

My new CI and its advanced technology was like having a new paint box with a full palette of colors that made my canvas come alive in ways I hadn't experienced before. I only used that processor alone for six months, though, so I hadn't reached my maximum potential with it. Pursuing perfection with one CI almost always meant doing well in the testing booth—single syllable words, sentences, in noise—with the assumption that the higher the scores, the closer I was to some elusive ideal. I now realize that it is impossible to achieve a true masterpiece with only one CI, old or new. That goal was a little naive.

The ultimate aim is not finding perfection in the testing booth. It is about behavior, not test scores—functioning at ease in the hearing world. That's why I won't be posting any more test scores here. I am still creating a masterpiece. But with two new paint boxes now and a brain to coordinate them, I'm not even sure what it's supposed to look like. With so many colors and combinations thrown into the mix, it sometimes feels more like finger painting than fine art!

Mapping sessions are still very much a part of this process and they too are starting to have a rhythm of their own. At my session last week, each ear was mapped individually, and then I listened with both processors on, trying to blend the sounds from both ears. They merged better this time than last, and that will presumably be the process—map/blend/adapt, then map/blend/adapt again and again—with hearing proficiency and associated behaviors subtly changing in the process.

This particular mapping and blending session evidently made a difference because I did notice some interesting behaviors emerge this week. I had occasion to participate in two group discussions— one with three people and one with four. These individuals did not know me, so they were not aware of my hearing loss. We were moving about in quiet settings, talking all the while, yet I could listen and hear—and function. At one point, one of them missed what was said, and I filled them in! I was with each group for about two hours, and during that time, I did not mention my hearing. I'm not even sure why except it didn't seem necessary. I did notice how well I was doing—I was navigating the casual conversation with markedly less stress. I've had similar encounters, of course, where there was no need to talk about my hearing, but never in social interactions of this duration. I guess this deserves the designation *bilateral moment*—a benchmark of behavior that could only have occurred using two ears.

I also attended a doll auction, one of my favorite things to do. I would usually sit up front to hear and see optimally. This time I discovered I could sit farther back, which I preferred, and still hear the auctioneer without looking. In fact, I was able to do a crossword puzzle while listening to the auction proceedings. I had never done this before, and it was heavenly! I felt a surge of confidence, being able to sit wherever I wanted and do whatever I pleased without being weighed down by hearing logistics.

Thinking about these and other experiences over the past several months—listening in noisy environments, turning to my name from a distance, the ease of casual conversations, turning to danger, not talking about my hearing, sitting wherever I please—these behaviors are literally coloring my personality. It is not at all like having one ear, where progress seemed to be absolute, measurable, and calculated. In essence, the masterpiece I am creating this time is more like an impressionist painting—a Renoir portrait, perhaps? The shades are subtle, they blend, you can't really see the image clearly unless you step back, and it takes a while to appreciate what you're looking at. The image that is emerging is someone who can hear even better than before—smiling, shining, confident—and *hearing impaired* continues to recede farther into the background.

EPILOGUE

E ven though my new ear is still adapting and both ears haven't
fully merged yet, I still sense that the mission here is complete.
The benefits of bilateral hearing described by the professionals have
come to fruition—generally better hearing, directionality, hearing
better in noise, and simply liking having two ears. It's time now to
stop and reflect.

The transformation that brought me to this point has, quite
honestly, been exhausting. Being thrust into twenty-four days of
isolating silence and then brought back to a world full of sound was
an education in itself. The contrast convinced me more than ever
that cochlear implants are a true miracle, allowing people who are
deaf to hear. That said, I now realize that hearing with one cochlear
implant is literally only half the story. The intricate interaction
between two ears and the brain enables representations of sound
that are often impossible with just one ear. The fact that bilateral
cochlear implants can replicate this two-ear/brain dynamic is a miracle in its own right!

And that brings me to my original question: Was this yearlong
odyssey just a series of random events or was it part of some grand
design? It is instructive to consider the issues covered in this book:
living with a degenerative hearing loss, the wonder of receiving a
cochlear implant and returning to the world of sound, the impact of
being thrust into total silence, improved functioning using current

cochlear implant processors, and the dynamics of listening with two ears. These chronicles have provided a comprehensive education about cochlear implants and deafness in the most graphic way possible—through my personal experience. Consider, as well, that receiving two new processors, implanted six months apart, allowed me to pinpoint whether better hearing was the result of improved technology or bilateral function. And, of course, this odyssey was also a personal transformation that allowed me to have current information and perspectives.

Reflect, too, on those instances that I've described as ironic, too perfect, or impeccably timed. They seem to have either guided my path or eased the burdens of this transformation in some way. To cite just a few examples: The FCC enacting telephone relay services exactly when I needed them; the picture of Helen Keller with her doll emerging after 120 years during the week my device failed; my cochlear implant failing at a CI support group meeting; the presence of "angels" at opportune moments, like Jody showing up "by chance" at my bilateral activation; the hospital workshop on bilateral cochlear implants scheduled exactly when I needed this information; the timely revision of my medical insurer's policies approving bilateral cochlear implants; that cryptic "Heavens to Betsy" crossword puzzle answer; the Yom Kippur shofar-blowing at the onset of my bilateral hearing; and of course, the recurring theme, "Someone to Watch Over Me."

Whatever one's thoughts about a grand design or divine intervention, the mission does seem to have been the production of this book, geared to educate about the impact of hearing loss and cochlear implants. The message is clear: Cochlear implants, which enable the deaf to hear, are true miracles of Biblical proportions.

And that is the message that needs to be heard.

HOW A COCHLEAR IMPLANT WORKS

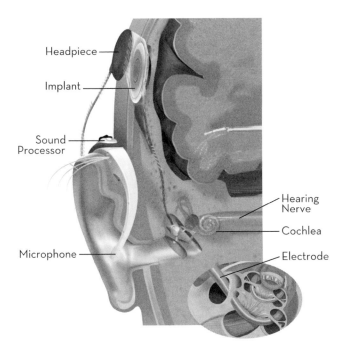

S ound waves enter the **MICROPHONE** located in the earhook of the external **SOUND PROCESSOR**. The **SOUND PROCESSOR** converts the electrical signal into a distinctive digital code that is programmed specifically to maximize each individual's sound and speech understanding.

Once processed, the electrically coded signal is sent up the thin cable to the **HEADPIECE** and is transmitted through the scalp via radio waves to the **IMPLANT**. The **HEADPIECE** is held in place by magnets.

The **IMPLANT** decodes the signal and delivers it to the array of **ELECTRODES** positioned deep within the **COCHLEA**.

The **ELECTRODES** bypass the damaged hair cells and directly stimulate the **HEARING NERVE** fibers within the **COCHLEA**.

Stimulation of the **HEARING NERVE** fibers causes electrical impulses to be delivered to the brain where they are interpreted as sound.

ACKNOWLEDGEMENTS

From the moment I began writing these chronicles, it was apparent that I was not alone in this odyssey. At every turn, there always seemed to be someone offering just the right words of encouragement or gesture of support. I am so grateful for every act of kindness, and want to recognize, with particular thanks, the following people:

My husband, Ira—for being there for me.

My children, Michael and Emily, and their spouses, Heatherlynn and James—for always seeming to know what to do to keep me going and smiling.

The dedicated professional staff at NYU Medical Center:
Dr. Thomas Roland—for his surgical skill and compassionate care.
Betsy Bromberg—the quintessential expert at mapping my ears.
Jody Gill—for holding my hand, both physically and metaphorically.

The Center for Hearing and Communication ("The League")—my lifeline over the years—whose dedicated, professional staff used every possible resource to keep me hearing and functioning.

The wonderful people at Advanced Bionics—for their caring and compassionate support.

Rabbi Peter Berg and Rabbi Ruth Zlotnick—for their spiritual support and invaluable guidance.

Andrea Grohman—for making me laugh when I should have been crying.

Karin Mango—for always encouraging my writing.

My friends at the Hearing Loss Association of America and the Hearing Loss Association of New Jersey—for their understanding and heartfelt encouragement on this journey.

My online friends and CI support network—available 24/7 with encouragement and advice.

MY LIFE HAS BEEN enriched by this experience, especially the outpouring of love and caring from so many.

INDEX